The Total Fat Cure:

Solving the Fat Trap

Laurens Maas
B.Sc.Ost, Dl.Hom. G.Os.C. & FBIH (UK)

Foreword by Dr. Robert Hempleman

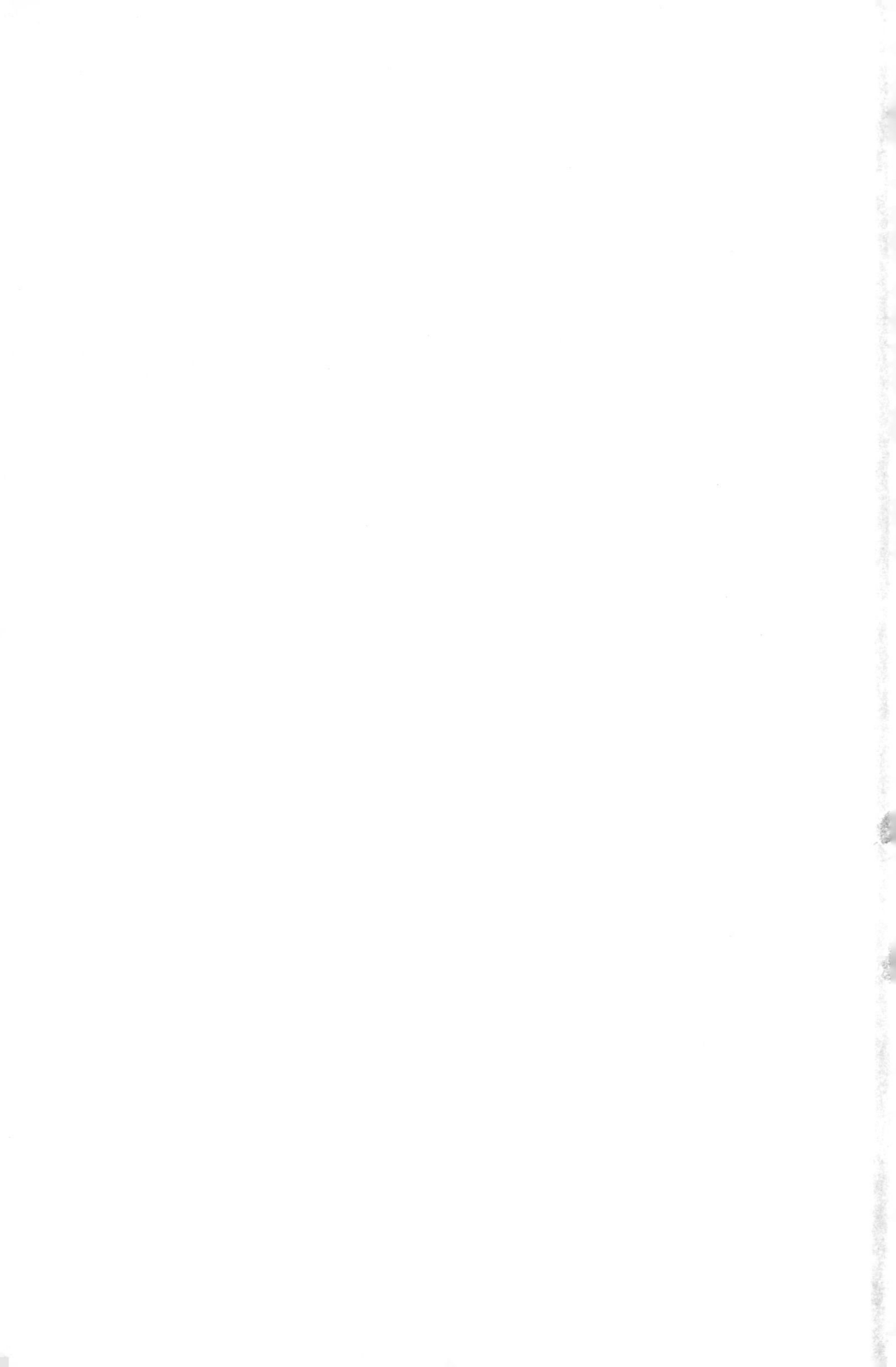

The Total Fat Cure:

Solving the Fat Trap

Laurens Maas
B.Sc.Ost, Dl.Hom. G.Os.C. & FBIH (UK)

Foreword by Dr. Robert Hempleman

Mill City Press, Minneapolis

Copyright © 2015 by Laurens Maas
www.themaasclinic.com

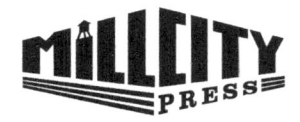

MILL CITY PRESS

Mill City Press, Inc.
322 First Avenue N, 5th floor
Minneapolis, MN 55401
612.455.2293
www.millcitypublishing.com

All rights reserved. No part of this publication may be reproduced, stored in a retrieval system, or transmitted, in any form or by any means, electronic, mechanical, photocopying, recording, or otherwise, without the prior written permission of the author.

Medical Disclaimer

All clinical material published by the author is for educational and informational purposes only. Readers are encouraged to confirm the holistic and medical information contained herein with other references and sources.

Patients and consumers should consult their physician or health-care provider before embarking on any health program, including the Total Fat Cure: Solving the Fat Trap. This raises a good opportunity to get some blood and hormone tests done while discussing the merits of this book.

The information contained herein is not intended to replace the medical advice offered by your physician. The author will not be liable for any direct, indirect, consequential, special, exemplary, or other damages arising there from.

ISBN-13: 978-1-63413-156-8
LCCN: 2014920495

Book design by James Arneson
Illustrations by Sarah Vieira
Edited by Laurens Maas
Image credit: Genova Diagnostic Labs

Printed in the United States of America

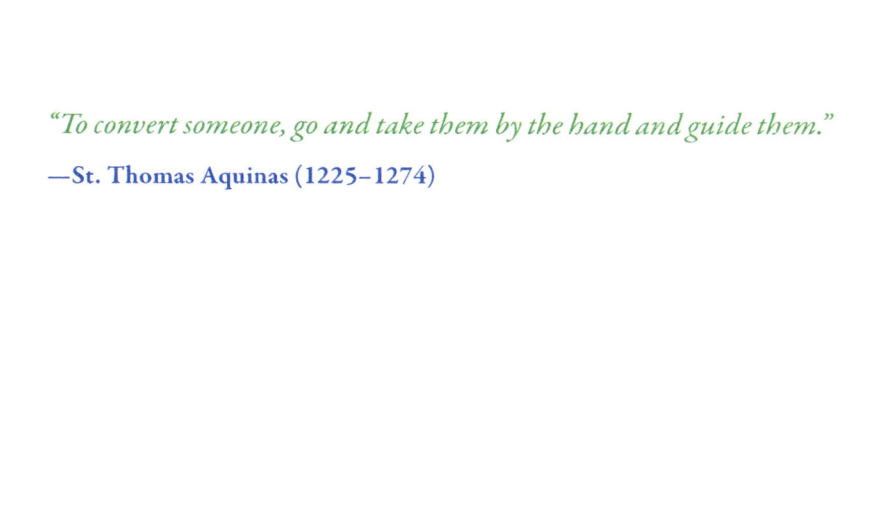

"To convert someone, go and take them by the hand and guide them."
—St. Thomas Aquinas (1225–1274)

Contents

Foreword	ix
Acknowledgments	xi
Introduction: The Fat Trap—Stress, How It Makes Humans Hungry, Tired, and Fat	xiii

THE PROBLEM — 1

Chapter 1	The Globesity Pandemic	3
Chapter 2	Chemicals, Antibiotics, Yeast, and Fungus Are Stressful	18
Chapter 3	Weight Gain and the Eight Fat Hormones	36

THE TESTING — 47

Chapter 4	Testing Your Eight Fat-Causing Hormones	49
Chapter 5	Testing Cortisol Levels	52
Chapter 6	Tracking Your Blood Sugars	73
Chapter 7	Testing for Estrogen Dominance	75
Chapter 8	Testing for Progesterone Deficiency	79
Chapter 9	Testing for Testosterone Deficiency	81
Chapter 10	Testing the Thyroid Gland	86
Chapter 11	Testing Your Leptin, Adiponectin, Ghrelin, and Melatonin Levels	91

THE SOLUTION — 93

Chapter 12	Controlling Your Eight Fat-Causing Hormones	95
Chapter 13	Creating Your Fat-Burning Plate	121

| **Chapter 14** | Strong Body | 135 |
| **Chapter 15** | Strong Mind | 149 |

THE KNOWLEDGE — 159

Glycemic Index of Selected Foods	161
Blood Chemistry Interpretation Charts	166
Blood Sugar Testing Chart	168

Appendix: Useful Contacts — 171

About the Author — 172

Foreword

If you Google "weight loss books," you have in excess of 208,000,000 results. This indicates the amount of literature published. Most books these days either *rehash* the same storyline from a flavor-of-the-month celebrity, or otherwise advocate a new approach that may work in the short term but ultimately may put the body into a degenerative state, e.g. protein-based diets that promote body acidity and lead to all sorts of problems.

So I first heard about osteopath/homeopath Mr. Laurens Maas about five years ago from a set of husband-and-wife patients who have since become good friends. The husband was suffering from Parkinson's and had been to Laurens for advice, guidance, and successful treatment. He has recovered substantially and leads a good life now. What particularly struck me was that here was a highly qualified complementary practitioner conducting wide-ranging established, analytical medical tests before using his broad knowledge to advise and treat his patients.

It is indeed *rare* these days to find practitioners using conventional medical tests, hormone levels, etc., as a basis for their approach/treatment. All too often well-meaning complementary practitioners (from many fields) recommend vitamins, minerals, and based on nothing but their own judgment. This is not the case with Mr. Laurens Maas, with his extensive training in functional medicine.

In this book, as a true holistic physician, Laurens Maas continues his scientific approach, focusing on weight loss, starting with conventional medical tests and then applying his very broad thinking and knowledge to providing the solution. He has found a combination of general lifestyle changes, low-dose bioidentical hormone therapy, recognized supplements, and two not-so-well-known herbs that form an effective weight-loss program. The theory behind this is easily and clearly explained step-by-step so that the reader can understand and go on to apply and use this knowledge.

It's not just about taking supplements, though. Just as important are the reduction of stress and the fitness of the mind and body. Here Laurens Maas once again has several chapters explaining different approaches and methods to gently ease you into a whole new experience.

In summary, this is not just about a new exercise or diet program but is a fully scientific and comprehensive fat-loss book covering the many different aspects that need to be addressed to achieve permanent weight loss healthily.

The successful reader will not only achieve weight loss but will undoubtedly have a whole new approach to and appreciation of life.

—Dr. Robert Hempleman, BDS (London), LDSRCS (UK)
Holistic Dental Practitioner

Acknowledgments

Thank you to my wife, Cathie, and my three children, Phoenix, Phoebe, and Cosmo; I am blessed to be with you all.

Many thanks to Dr. Dicken Weatherby, ND; Dr. Dan Kalish, DC; Dr. Patrick Hanaway, MD, head of Genova Labs; Dr. Bruce Shelton, MD, DiHom; Dr. Joseph Mercola, DO; Steve Denk at BioMedX Chicago; Dr. Richard Bandler and John La Valle for the knowledge and guidance they shared with me and imparted so willingly to make humanity healthier on many levels. I have found all of them to be a constant source of inspiration. They have all influenced my medical philosophy positively. Thank you to Genova Labs USA for allowing me to use some of their hormone graphs.

Also a thank you to Dr. Robert Hempleman for writing the foreword to the book. We think clearly along the same lines, as he was witness to a close friend and patient's recovery using the same methods outlined in this book and my others. Biological dentistry holds hands with Functional Diagnostic Medicine in the key principles.

Thank you also to a multitude of my diabetic, overweight, and obese patients who helped me uncover, through careful observation and testing, how to really get humans to lose weight. Thank you for trusting me with my requests for good hormone testing, stool analysis, and patient application of the natural hormones to get the body that became slimmer and slimmer each week, each month, and each year. Thank you for allowing me to monitor your progress and for sharing your experiences with me. Without you I would not be the physician I am today.

I also have enormous gratitude to a dear patient and friend. I would like to thank Sarah-Jayne Vieira for all her professionalism, as she provided enormous support in the final push to get the book complete with updated images and final edits. A very grateful thank you.

—Laurens, 2014

Introduction

The Fat Trap—Stress, How It Makes Humans Hungry, Tired, and Fat

Most people never think that their stress levels could be making them hungry, tired, fat, and overweight. It's a relatively new theory about stress, weight gain, and obesity[1] in mammals, and yet time after time, over twenty years in practice, when I see my human patients correct their stress levels, balance their hormones, start to sleep well (eight hours), eat a good diet, and have regular moderate exercise, they all lose weight and create a self-healing response within the body.

Modern fast, processed food is stressful, devoid of essential vitamins and antioxidants, and is a form of undernutrition[2] that causes metabolic pressure on many hormone systems through deficiency, which in turn compensate by making us store *more fat* in the future. Certain processed Frankenfoods are programmed to make us hungry and fat (to make more sales). The processed-food industry creates meals that make you hungrier[3]. Hunger creates stress, sleep issues, and further hunger, and thus more sales eventually. Fast-food manufacturers and processed-food corporations want to make millions of sales, so what better than to make a food that is addictive and makes the consumer want more because the

---

1   Jeffrey M. Friedman and Jeffrey L. Halaas, "Leptin and the regulation of body weight in mammals," *Nature* 395.6704 (1998): 763–770.

2   P. N. Wilson and D. F. Osbourn, "Compensatory growth after undernutrition in mammals and birds," *Biological Reviews* 35.3 (1960): 324–361.

3   Susan B. Roberts, "High-Glycemic Index Foods, Hunger, and Obesity: Is There a Connection?"" *Nutrition Reviews* 58.6 (2000): 163–169.

actual food creates hunger. Crazy weight gain is the result. It's a program within the food.

The difficulty for all overweight and obese people, and what they don't realize, yet feel regularly, is that their own brains send excessive *hunger* signals to their stomachs, making them want to eat a lot of the time. This is the Fat Trap. Cheap carbs are stressful, and they give people a sugar "high" that makes them hungry and causes them to eat more of the same addictive, stress-inducing foods.

During stress and anxiety, there are eight hormones within our bodies that can go out of balance. The more stressed a person is, the greater the amount of damage to the hormone systems of the body that regulate body fat, which I have seen in clinical practice and is backed by a lot of references. Unfortunately a lot of MDs don't get taught Functional Medicine, and as such they usually see weight gain as a result of too many carbs and not enough exercise. It's a very old-fashioned view.

The secret to satisfying weight loss, which I see in my overweight patients, is to figure how many of the actual eight hormones are out of balance and to return them back to optimal levels using the techniques and lifestyle suggestions outlined in this book. Once that happens, the metabolism switches back on, the weight comes off, and health returns to your body and mind, as it's a twofold journey.

The two slimming hormones that would normally be able to stop the massive hunger response (leptin and adiponectin) have been damaged through chronic stress and inflammation[4]. For example, even if the stress was as simple as eating processed/fast food regularly, that cheap, nasty food is actually stressful because it is genetically modified object GMO, likely to contain synthetic hormone–laced products, and has inadequate minerals. Or the

---

[4] Mark L. Heiman et al, "Leptin inhibition of the hypothalamic-pituitary-adrenal axis in response to stress," *Endocrinology* 138.9 (1997): 3859–3863.

stress event could have been a really bad physically damaging injury from the past—being shot, car accident, nasty divorce, or even mental stress from studying for a PhD! Overwhelming stress hurts our hormones and our metabolism.

Most people these days, when they *think* of weight loss and burning fat, they automatically think dieting, extreme exercise and food deprivation, and the amount or lack of willpower to achieve their desired goals. Food deprivation and intense exercise, by the way, is stressful, so that approach is doomed to cause more weight gain if the person is already burnt-out. We need to eat to create energy, and that comes from choosing good quality foods, minerals and balanced hormones.

However, I am here to tell you in this introduction that people who are naturally slim and muscular, who have abundant energy and are happy, don't really ever think about dieting and *extreme* exercise. They just have a good lifestyle and great hormone levels that keep them in a state of balance. They can build fat and break it down just as fast. Their systems of appetite control—that is, the communication between their brains and their adrenal and thyroid glands and between the quantity of fat reserves and their stomach—remain balanced even if they eat fat, sugar, and carbs. So what throws off the balance of fat-burning and fat-building hormones?

In simple words, it is *stress and strain of modern life.* Really simple, but in actuality the pressure affects many hormones *negatively* and the stress can come from many levels, and it results in an insatiable hunger, a gnawing inside. That hunger reflex is what causes the programmed self-sabotage while on a low-carb diet. Almost every weight-loss diet is doomed to fail through self-sabotage. It's the hunger signal, created by a warped brain influenced by Frankenfoods, emotional stress, or even parasite and allergy stressors.

FAT & WEIGHT GAIN

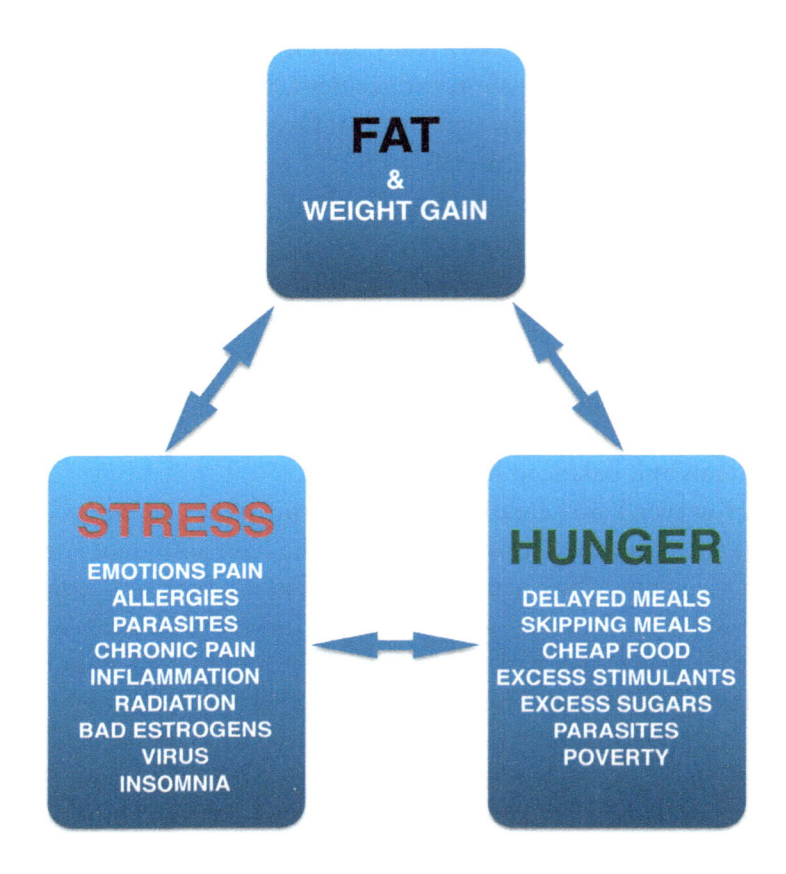

STRESS
EMOTIONS PAIN
ALLERGIES
PARASITES
CHRONIC PAIN
INFLAMMATION
RADIATION
BAD ESTROGENS
VIRUS
INSOMNIA

HUNGER
DELAYED MEALS
SKIPPING MEALS
CHEAP FOOD
EXCESS STIMULANTS
EXCESS SUGARS
PARASITES
POVERTY

The Fat Trap Triangle—Stress, Hunger, and Fat.

Stress Exists on Many Levels

Stress is such a general term, and most of the time it's not actually understood or treated properly. Most people suffer from emotional stress (e.g., anger, frustration, despair, watching horror movies), dietary stress (e.g., food allergies, food poisoning, mercury in fish/dental fillings), and pain and hidden sources of inflammation (e.g., radiation, parasites, and pharmaceuticals).

Stressful lifestyles can create abnormal hunger signals, and these could come from skipping or delaying meals too often, chronic parasites, heavy metals and radiation, and cheap processed foods. Divorce can be stressful and makes those involved fatter because of the intense emotional stress. High-ranking politicians slowly become fatter over their careers. Physical trauma to the body can also cause weight gain weeks or months later. Being mauled by an animal is stressfull, and therefore being mauled internally by a silent parasite infection is even more stressful because one can't run away from the parasite if it's inside you. Parasites can cause weight gain.

All these different types of stress can trigger your body to go into fat-storage mode, mainly through the mechanism of the eight key hormones. There is a connection between emotional glands in our brain (hypothalamus and pituitary) and our adrenal stress and thyroid glands. This connection is called the HPAT axis—the Hypothalamic-Pituitary-Adrenal-Thyroid axis—a neuroendocrine connection that marries the emotions of the brain with the adrenal and thyroid glands and wake/sleep cycles.

When stressed, cortisol—a hormone that's needed to deal with any stress—causes the blood sugar to rise, which in turn creates inflammation that then blocks our ability to burn fat[5] via a distorted HPAT axis[6]. When a person is stressed, the body thinks it is going to run out of food. This is an ancestral response, because the first stressors programmed into us in early human life were from emotional separation, starvation and physical pain and injury.

Fat is the body's security blanket against starvation stress, but when people experience negative emotions,[7] trauma, parasites, and allergies, they will gain weight eventually because cortisol

---

5 Mark L. Heiman et al, "Leptin inhibition of the hypothalamic-pituitary-adrenal axis in response to stress," *Endocrinology* 138.9 (1997): 3859–3863.

6 Wisse, Brent E., and Michael W. Schwartz. "Does hypothalamic inflammation cause obesity?." *Cell metabolism* 10.4 (2009): 241-242.

7 Richard S. Lazarus, Emotion and Adaptation, (New York: Oxford University Press, pg 29-68, 1991),

creates sugar swings. The delicate connection between the brain and the glands of the body somehow short-circuits, a progressive stress burnout that stimulates fat cells to increase in size, fueling the process with further daily hunger signals.

The world is full of sorrow and pain; the sad reality is that *stress* affects us on several levels in a "modern society." These levels include psychological and emotional issues as well as dietary stress and pain/hidden inflammation stress[8].

The importance for you as the reader is to understand that the HPAT axis gets damaged through emotional, dietary, and pain stress and trauma. The good news is that this delicate connection can be repaired through a good, wholesome low-stress lifestyle that rebuilds the adrenals and their connectivity to the HPAT axis; regular sleep, regular balanced meals, and good emotions all play their part in repairing this connection.

Doctors often prescribe sleeping pills, cholesterol drugs, tranquilizers, painkillers, heart medications, and headache tablets, but they do not address the cause of individuals' *stress* but only the symptoms—such as insomnia, weight gain, high blood pressure, anxiety, acute pain, depression, and chronic pain. Allow me to quote from an article in *Life Extension*[9] magazine from December 2007 about the holistic-minded Dr. Edward Lichten, MD FACS, about his perspective on the orthodox medical establishment's view on stress and the adrenals:

> Many chronic illnesses can be traced back to adrenal malfunction, yet mainstream medicine does not even consider this part of the anatomy when prescribing treatments. The chronic fatigue and stress that so many people are stricken with often emanates from

---

[8] Dr. Dan Kalish, Institute Course Material in Functional Medicine. San Diego, CA: Physician training material 2011

[9] Dale Kiefer, "The Benefits of Bio-Identical Hormones," Life Extension December 2007. This provides an overview of Dr. Edward Licthen's (MD FACS)' book *The Textbook of Bio-Identical Hormones*.

the adrenals. Dr. Lichten has developed protocols to diagnose and treat these conditions that the medical establishment has all but ignored even though the natural hormones needed were long ago discovered and documented in the published medical literature to be effective.

In fact, most MDs will completely ignore their patients' stress, because unfortunately they are not taught adrenal recovery programs in medical school. Very few MDs know how to advise on stress management, and even fewer would know how to treat the effects of stress naturally using diet and lifestyle changes and bioidentical hormones. There are a few MDs, however, who have recognized how important the adrenal hormones role is in treating diseases and reestablishment of normal metabolism, but these are *extreme* adrenal diseases such as Addison's disease and Cushing's syndrome, and they usually prescribe synthetic hormones that have life-saving properties but negative side effects too (diabetes, weight gain, osteoporosis, weak tissues etc). Most people with acute stress (hyperadrenia) and adrenal burn-out (hypoadrenia) can easily recover using natural hormones, diet and lifestyle.

They might recognize that their patients are stressed, but how to treat them with adrenal support and lifestyle and diet changes is beyond most. Moreover, continually treating the symptoms[10] causes even more stress to the body, because it becomes loaded with a set of man-made chemicals that are unnatural to the body, and the body finds the drug approach stressful on a physiological level that is already out of balance. The drugs force the body to change rather than rebalancing the systems naturally. Stress again (pharmacological).

---

10   Maclaren, W. R., and D. E. Frank. "Continuous steroid hormone treatment of chronic asthma. I. Cortisone and hydrocortisone." *Annals of allergy* 14.2 (1956): 183.

Stress, Hunger, and Fat Domino Effect

When stress happens, cortisol, a glucocorticosteroid hormone, works with insulin to adjust the blood-sugar levels. If cortisol goes high from a stressor(s), so does blood sugar, and repeated high blood sugar causes the body to store fat. Stress will prompt a fat-causing *effect* from the high Cortisol/ high blood sugar (and also adrenalin) as it rises in the blood, to help cope with the stressor(s).

The dominoe effect is that if cortisol rises, estrogen rises and testosterone will fall, thereby making people lose their muscle density and become flabby. The loss of testosterone[11] in men is a marker for development of type 2 (T2) diabetes. The inner symptoms of male andropause include insulin resistance, which can lead to diabetes, weight gain, depression, atherosclerosis, and fatigue. In women there are further symptoms of poor muscle tone, depression, anxiety, joint problems, frigidity and atherosclerosis.

This also explains why when people try to lose weight with diet and excessive exercise, it will traditionally fail in the long term, because *overtraining in itself*, which a lot of overweight people tend to do to get the weight off, can "hurt" the body (its testosterone levels fall, muscle weakness and low libido set in, etc.), and this becomes another stressor. No pain, no gain. Really? I don't think so, well not for burn-out patients anyway.

This observation also explains why when people go on a sunny holiday and they eat the same, and they seem to lose weight without thinking about it. Because they are *finally* relaxing. The relaxation effect via the sunny vitamin D pathway, lowers cortisol and allows the testosterone levels to rise. It also explains why humans, when they tan, also get horny, and they start to burn

---

[11] M. Rabijewski, J. Kozakowski, and W. Zgliczyski. "The relationship between Testosterone concentrations, Insulin resistance and visceral obesity in elderly men." *Endkrynol Pol.* 56 (6) (2005): 897–903.

fat (with a balanced diet). If tanning doesn't create an increase in libido within you, then this might be an indicator that one may be low in testosterone. Also before embarking on this weight loss lifestyle, please make sure you have optimal Vitamin D (25 Hydroxy) levels between 50-70 ng/ml[12]. This is a very important vitamin and can be taken either through tanning with regular sunshine or Vit D supplements.

If your testosterone (male or female) fails to reach optimal levels, then adding in a bioidentical testosterone will achieve great results[13] in reversing T2 diabetes (men), improving libido, muscle mass, confidence, and weight loss. Progesterone is also a fat burner, and women must have higher levels in order to lose weight. Stress lowers our sex hormones. Later in the book I will tell you how you can fix those whacky hormones.

When the body is stressed, one of the symptoms is weight gain; other symptoms can be headaches, insomnia, mood swings, and chronic fatigue. There are a few who, when stressed, will lose a lot of weight and become anorexic (less than 10 percent; this is the minority). If one connects the dots, many chronic illnesses can be sourced to chronic adrenal and thyroid problems from stressful diets and lifestyles, but conventional medicine never takes this into consideration when prescribing drugs to patients.

So many people are stricken with weight gain, chronic fatigue, diabetes, and immune disorders, and over and over again I see it relates to hormone dysfunction in my patients within the clinic. Low hormones create diseases[14].

---

12   Dr.J.Mercola DO, http://articles.mercola.com/sites/articles/archive/2011/11/21/how-to-get-your-vitamin-d-to-healthy-ranges.aspx

13   Rabijewski M, Kozakowski J, Zgliczyski W. The relationship between testosterone and dehydroepiandrosterone sulfate concentrations, insulin resistance and visceral obesity in elderly men. *Endokrynol Pol*. 2005 Nov-Dec;56(6):897-903

14   Howard, James Michael. "Common factor of cancer and the metabolic syndrome may be low DHEA." *Annals of epidemiology* 17, no. 4 (2007): 270.

To lose weight one has to change one's mind-set and lifestyle for the better and to create the lifestyle that helps the hormones come back into balance and *stay* in balance. It's what this book is about.

> **FACT: Worldwide there are now one billion overweight adults and three hundred million obese people. There are a lot of stressed people out in the world.**

Guess which nations lead the chubby consensus[15]? Micronesia and Tonga, followed by the USA. Britain ranks tenth. Across the Atlantic in the USA, Americans rule the world with a figure of about 55 percent of citizens being overweight[16] or obese[17]. This data is a little old but clearly points out that the trend of weight gain and obesity is still rising. There is a huge wave of obesity affecting millions of innocent humans who haven't known how to fix it, until now.

Cortisol & Stress, Parasites, Allergies, and Weight Gain

Stress causes a lot of diseases. Diseases associated with cortisol dysfunction are as follows: food allergies[18]; anorexia[19] ; ear, nose, and

---

15   http://www.telegraph.co.uk/earth/earthnews/9345086/The-worlds-fattest-countries-how-do-you-compare.html

16   Federal Obesity Clinical Guidelines; 6/1998 National heart Lung and Blood Inst. / National Inst. Diabetes, Digestive and Kidney disease. http://www.nhlbi.nih.gov/guidelines/obesity/ob_gdlns.pdf

17   http://www.huffingtonpost.com/2012/02/22/obesity-rates-rising-developed-fattest-world_n_1294212.html

18   L. Chatzi, M. Torrent, I. Romieu et al, "Diet, wheeze, and atopy in school children in Menorca, Spain," *Pediatr Allergy Immunol* 18(6) (2007): 480–485.

19   Peter Doerr et al, "Relationship between weight gain and hypothalamic pituitary adrenal function in patients with anorexia nervosa." *Journal of Steroid Biochemistry* 13.5 (1980): 529–537.

throat allergies; asthma[20]; infections; obesity[21]; schizophrenia[22]; osteoporosis; anxiety; depression[23]; chronic fatigue[24]; diabetes[25]; cardiovascular diseases[26]; and breast cancer[27].

Parasites, bacteria, yeast, and allergies will raise cortisol levels and lower DHEA levels. Parasites, bacteria, yeast, and allergies are stressful, right? Most overweight and fat people unknowingly have chronic bacterial infections, which can induce their obesity[28]. One in particular has been clearly linked with weight gain, and it's called Enterobacter cloacae B29[29]. Killing the bacterial overgrowth

---

20 S. Fitzpatrick, R. Joks, and J. I. Silverberg, "Obesity is associated with increased asthma severity and exacerbations, and increased serum immunoglobulin E in inner-city adults," *Clinical & Expermental Allergy*, (2011).

21 Ibid 57

22 Michael Ritsner et al, "Elevation of the cortisol/dehydroepiandrosterone ratio in schizophrenia patients," *European Neuropsychopharmacology* 14.4 (2004): 267–273.

23 Heather M. Burke et al, "Depression and cortisol responses to psychological stress: a meta-analysis," *Psychoneuroendocrinology* 30.9 (2005): 846–856.

24 Paul Strickland et al, "A comparison of salivary cortisol in chronic fatigue syndrome, community depression and healthy controls," *Journal of Affective Disorders* 47.1 (1998): 191–194.

25 Robert C. Andrews and Brian R. Walker, "Glucocorticoids and insulin resistance: old hormones, new targets," *Clinical Science* 96 (1999): 513–523.

26 P. Björntorp, "Visceral fat accumulation: the missing link between psychosocial factors and cardiovascular disease?" *Journal of Internal Medicine* 230.3 (1991): 195–201.

27 Dean G. Cruess et al, "Cognitive-behavioral stress management reduces serum cortisol by enhancing benefit finding among women being treated for early stage breast cancer," *Psychosomatic Medicine* 62.3 (2000): 304–308.

28 Matej Bajzer & Randy J. Seeley, "Physiology: Obesity and gut flora," *Nature* 444 (21 December 2006): 1009–1010. | doi:10.1038/4441009a; Published online 21 December 2006

29 "An opportunistic pathogen isolated from the gut of an obese human causes obesity in germfree mice," *The ISME Journal*. December 13, 2012. doi:10.1038. ISSN 1751-7362. Retrieved December 18, 2012 source :.http://www.nature.com/ismej/journal/v7/n4/full/ismej2012153a.html

induces serious weight loss. Parasites, too, can cause weight gain, according to many scientists[30]. Parasites are like tigers attacking us from inside, and the problem is that we can't run away from the gut tiger, so the stress keeps getting worse as the parasite grows. A lot of my overweight patients have parasites, and sometimes there are several within the gut, layer after layer, proved by repeated stool testing.

People also can mistakenly consume foods they're allergic to, sometimes on a daily basis. When this happens, your body responds with stress[31], which triggers the release of cortisol[32], and this in turn screws up the blood's sugar levels and makes us put on weight.

> **KEY POINT: Cortisol is a *glucocorticosteroid*, and when it is secreted during any stress (psychological, physical, and physiological), the blood sugar will be forced to rise, and that starts a chain reaction of a hunger, stress, tired, and fat effect.**

This cortisol release upsets the regulation of sugars because "stress" causes the body to release more sugar to the muscles when they enter the flight, or fright, or fight mode. Evolution said that if you are going to run from an attacking animal, you'll need some instant fuel (sugar) to get the leg muscles to start moving faster. Blood sugar rises quickly when we get angry, upset, and tense, and the thing is, we can't run away from the angry emotional bear because it's inside us. The angry blood sugar stays in the blood, creating inflammation. Poor sleep, too, will cause sugars to rise from the stress of having not slept properly.

As blood-sugar levels repeatedly rise up and down erratically, like a roller coaster, the pancreas will also grow tired over time, and

---

30   http://undergroundhealthreporter.com/causes-of-obesity#axzz2rYgnaeB0

31   F. Stenius, M. Borres, and M. Bottai et al, "Salivary cortisolcortisol levels and allergy in children: the ALADDIN birth cohort," *Journal of Allergy Clinical Immunology* 128(6) (2011): 1335–1339.

32   A. Buske-Kirschbaum, "cortisolcortisol responses to stress in allergic children: interaction with the immune response," *Neuro-immunomodulation* 16(5) (2009): 325–332.

its ability to handle sugars goes into decline. This sets the stage for diabetes and weight gain. Allergies (also known as antigens) create antibodies within the blood. Antibodies are the body's response to allergies so it can recognize the difference between self and nonself. Experiencing an allergy attack is stressful.

While your body is creating antibodies against parasites, food allergies, and toxins, you're also making reactive chemical substances such as histamines, cytokines, lymphokines, and interferon. These substances act like hormones and as such create dramatic effects on physiology, which can have profound effects on the human nervous system, glandular systems of the thyroid and adrenals, and immune system. Many of these effects are fat cell build up, chronic fatigue and low energy levels.

Parasites, food, and environmental toxins have been connected to a wide range of medical conditions from mild symptoms of gastric reflux to very serious diseases such as heart diseases and cancer. Allergies also have been openly associated with migraines, depression, arthritis, and chronic fatigue immunodeficiency syndrome.

Common Parasites Symptoms
1. Chronic allergies
2. Dark circles under eyes
3. Gas
4. Bloating
5. Belching
6. Chronic constipation, IBS
7. Diarrhea, IBS
8. Burning anus
9. Itchy anus
10. Difficulty losing weight
11. Difficulty gaining weight
12. Chronic fatigue
13. Depression

14. ADD
15. ADHD
16. Colitis (Crohn's/ Ulcerative)

American Apple Body Shape

Most people in America have the same body shape. The apple body shape has become the norm in America, with many people carrying the same spare tire around their midsections. This is a quote from the National Institute of Health Guidelines[33]:

> An estimated 97 million adults in the United States are overweight or obese, a condition that substantially raises their risk of morbidity from hypertension, dyslipidemia, type 2 diabetes, coronary heart disease, stroke, gallbladder disease, osteoarthritis, sleep apnea and respiratory problems, and endometrial, breast, prostate, and colon cancers. Higher body weights are also associated with increases in all-cause mortality. Obese individuals may also suffer from social stigmatization and discrimination. As a major contributor to preventive death in the United States today, overweight and obesity pose a major public health challenge.

I was rudely awakened to these figures when I traveled with my family to Orlando to do the Disney trip with the kids. I had been to the same water park thirty-one years before and was not witness to so many obese people then!

What could have happened in thirty years that could contribute to such exaggerated weight gain?

At Disney, I overheard a couple that collectively weighed about seven hundred pounds talking about a new diet pill, whilst waiting in a long line for a water ride. I heard them say this new "magic pill" on the market would help them to lose weight without exercising

---

[33] Clinical Guidelines on the Identification, Evaluation, and Treatment of Overweight and Obesity in Adults: *The Evidence Report* https://www.nhlbi.nih.gov/guidelines/obesity/ob_gdlns.htm

or changing their diet. They were excited about not having to do any work for their beautiful new bodies.

My conclusion, as I was standing in the queues of the various rides with many average overweight Americans, was that *they themselves had really no idea* how they got that way, as I eavesdropped on the overweight couples chatting about fat. They gave their opinions on gastric constriction bands and liposuction, who had tried what food or pill, how it had failed, and the whole nine yards. From a professional perspective, it was enlightening.

They did not talk once about the issues of stressful lifestyles, parasites, and allergic diets laced with sugar and synthetic hormones that program people to get hungry and fat. They just didn't know, in an innocent kind of way, while waiting in the queue for the water ride, what factors were making them fatter each year. In hindsight, that trip concretized my understanding about obesity and weight issues and how they fundamentally relate to excess estrogens in the food chain, environment, and copious amounts of stressful carbohydrate-based meals loaded with yeast and cheap sugars.

In the spirit of treating symptoms, Americans lead the world in bariatric surgery, gastric constriction bands , and liposuction with early mortality[34] and high failure rates[35],[36]. They live and eat just like everybody else but have the highest rates of obesity. What they don't know is that within their environment is an invisible

---

34 David R. Flum et al, "Early mortality among Medicare beneficiaries undergoing bariatric surgical procedures," JAMA: *The Journal of the American Medical Association* 294.15 (2005): 1903–1908.

35 Eric J. DeMaria et al, "High failure rate after laparoscopic adjustable silicone gastric banding for treatment of morbid obesity," *Annals of Surgery* 233.6 (2001): 809.

36 V. Giusti MD, PD, "A 10-year experience with laparoscopic gastric banding for morbid obesity: high long-term complication and failure rates," *Obesity Surgery* 16.7 (2006): 829–835.

blanket of yeasts, estrogens, and xenoestrogens causing them to crave sugars and get fat[37] over many decades.

So what is responsible for the sharp increase in being overweight and obese? Well, according to the National Institute of Health, it is multifactorial[38]: Obesity is a complex, multifactorial chronic disease that develops from an interaction of genotype and the environment. Our understanding of how and why obesity develops is incomplete, but involves the integration of social, behavioral, cultural, physiological, metabolic, and genetic factors.

It's going to take some learning about how our past and present stressful lifestyles, the amount of sugar we consume, and how the sugars and hormones interact in our bodies cause massive weight gain. It's going to take some application and eventually a measure of *habit gravity* that will lead you to success. When science is properly applied, it can transform your body and mind for the better, and that will extend your life span.

Therein lies the miracle. The "miracle" is that your body has the power to heal itself. Self-healing is key, and what you are doing with this book is finding "your way" out of your fat puzzle. There are eight hormones that could potentially go out of whack. You will want to use the information in this book to tell you which hormones need to be boosted.

Losing weight may not only help control diseases but also reduces the risk of morbidity from hypertension; dyslipidemia; type 2 diabetes; coronary heart disease; stroke; gallbladder disease; osteoarthritis; sleep apnea and respiratory problems; and endometrial, breast, prostate, and colon cancers[39].

---

37   Kobayashi-Hattori, Kazuo, Chidozie J. Amuzie, Brenna M. Flannery, and James J. Pestka. "Body composition and hormonal effects following exposure to mycotoxin deoxynivalenol in the high-fat diet-induced obese mouse." *Molecular nutrition & food research* 55, no. 7 (2011): 1070-1078.

38   Ibid 33

39   Federal Obesity Clinical Guidelines; 6/1998 National heart Lung and Blood Inst. / National Inst. Diabetes, Digestive and Kidney disease. http://www.nhlbi.nih.gov/guidelines/obesity/ob_gdlns.pdf

If you think those pharmaceutical pills are *the real ticket* to a long and happy life, then you will end up truly discontented in the end. So try a scientific, natural way that works by aiding the body, and figure out which of the eight key hormones need balancing and fuse that with the diet recommendations for metabolic type and *paleo* blood-type proteins, and then you will see and feel the changes that you want.

The Fat Trap is the stress, hunger, tired, and fat triangle. This book will tell you how you got into the trap, and it tells you how to get out of the trap by understanding which of the eight hormones need to be tweaked, and it couples this with an ancestral and scientific diet plan.

THE PROBLEM

Chapter 1

The Globesity Pandemic

From this point on, *you* as the weight-loss reader need to know about some of the factors that you are up against. There is a huge tidal wave of obesity and diabetes sweeping the world. In this chapter, you will learn about the globesity pandemic, how our food chain has been impacted, and how, as a solution, we can turn toward our ancestral diets to help our genes recover.

Just the Facts, Ma'am!

A reporter at the World Health Organization (WHO) originally coined the word *globesity*. He stated in his 2001 report that there was a serious obesity epidemic facing the globe[1].

Here are some earth-shattering facts disclosed by the WHO in 2008[2]:

- 61 percent of Americans are overweight and 26 percent are obese.
- There are more than one billion overweight adults worldwide.
- There are more than three hundred million obese humans worldwide (2005).
- Obesity is proven to lead to other diseases, e.g. diabetes, heart disease, high blood pressure, and cancer.
- Weight gain is directly proportionate to increased eating of fast food, carbs, fats, and sugars and reduced physical activity.

---

1 http://www.macmillandictionaries.com/MED-Magazine/February2008/49-New-Word.htm

2 http://www.who.int/research/en/

- Overweight and obese individuals will die early.
- Childhood obesity is already an epidemic.

This may be facing America right now, but within the next decade, other first-, second-, and third-world countries will be experiencing the same crisis. Globesity is now more of a problem than malnutrition and famine. In 2002 the WHO released another report about diet and chronic disease. The report highlighted the immediacy of the pandemic and lamented that without serious government intervention, the problem would clearly get worse. Unfortunately, it already has.

The report also includes advice on changing the diet of overweight and obese individuals by:

- Reducing energy-rich foods high in saturated fat and sugar
- Cutting the amount of salt in the diet
- Increasing the amount of fresh fruit and vegetables in the diet
- Undertaking moderate-intensity physical activity for at least an hour a day

Okay, this report has good instructions, but we need to know a bit more about "what" else is "out there" that can cause us to get fat in the first place. Let me enlighten you.

The Modern Disease of Central Obesity

In the wake of Dr. Atkins, Dr. Arthur Agatston, MD[3], renowned cardiologist and author of *The South Beach Diet*, believes that abdominal fat is different and more dangerous than fat anywhere else in the body. Unlike fat directly under the skin, belly fat, which adheres to the organs, is linked to increases in a blood marker called C-reactive protein (CRP) and other markers of inflammation (homocysteine) that can lead to heart disease. CRP is linked to leptin resistance.

---

3 http://en.wikipedia.org/wiki/Arthur_Agatston

Agatston has achieved *great success* with patients on the South Beach Diet, and this is testament to the power of choosing the correct carbs, fats, and proteins more carefully, bearing in mind that insulin or sugar issues are directly related to *heart problems and weight gain*.

Conclusion: A famous US cardiologist basically saying that bad, unhealthy carbs can cause heart disease, diabetes, and fat storage. Bad carbs create fat cells and disease.

However, Agatston's theory is at best a "restricted carb"–based diet approach; it clearly works in some people, however it overlooks the WHO position that obesity and heart disease, as well as cancer, are related to mycotoxins in our food and environment. A popular fungus that we as humans consume regularly is yeast—in Brie, Camembert, bread, beer, other fermented beverages, smoked meats, etc. These yeasty foods are linked to heart disease, obesity, and cancer as proven by several MDs at the World Health Organization. Antibiotics made from fungal extracts create yeast infections, and the WHO has stated that antibiotics can cause cancer.

Professsor Costantini of the WHO showed that yeast obesity, and particularly abdominal obesity[4], is linked to ischemic heart disease, glucose intolerance, higher cholesterol, and hypertension, and these are all diseases associated with consumption of yeast-based beverages such as beer and wine[5]. Beer is a yeast-fermented beverage made from mycotoxins. Consuming any mycotoxins (including yeast/candida) causes massive stress on the liver's detoxification organs, thereby raising cortisol/CRP and inducing leptin resistance.

---

4 A. V. Costantini, Fungalbionics Series; Etiology and Prevention of Atherosclerosis. Johann Freidrich Oberlin Verlag. Freiburg, Germany. 1998/99. Chp 9 pg 47-49

5 Costantini, AV, Fungalbionics Series; Etiology and Prevention of Atherosclerosis. Johann Freidrich Oberlin Verlag. Freiburg, Germany. 1998/99. Chp 1, pg 9-10

Yeast is a major cause of heart disease and diabetes[6] because it is toxic to the body. As reported in my first book, *The Hidden Cure*, when you go antifungal you reduce your blood pressure and cholesterol, improve your heart function, and lose weight more readily though better glucose control via diet/supplements, eradication of yeast, and positive lifestyle changes.

You certainly don't have to be a drinker to get fat and diabetic. Dietary yeast is used in the fattening of pigs and cows[7], which also causes them to have higher milk yields. When yeast is given to these animals in their feed, they gain weight faster. Yeast causes more intense fat-cell growth and causes uric acid[8] to build up within the body tissues. As you will learn, uric acid (in the appendix), causes inflammation, pickles the pancreas and the immune system, as is highly toxic and will induce diabetes[9], kidney diseases[10], and leukemia. Clear proof that long-term yeast kills mammals slowly. Yeast is toxic, but it makes food taste better, and humans can become addicted to it.

Pig and cattle farmers have a significant investment in their livestock. In order to protect their living inventory, farmers routinely place the animals on antibiotics and yeast cultures. These prevent secondary infections in the animals and help a farmer reduce his losses. Farmers "have to" do this because their insurance

---

6   L. Maas B.Sc. Ost, Dl.Hom. The Hidden Cure. Wheatmark Pub. Chp. 5 pg 61. 2009

7   Jon Hughes & Pat Thomas, BLT Sandwich; The Big Lifestyle Trade-off, Ecologist Magazine, 22nd September, 2006

8   Richard J. Johnson, M.D., and Bruce A. Rideout, D.V.M., Ph.D. Uric Acid and Diet — Insights into the Epidemic of Cardiovascular Disease. Richard J. Johnson, M.D., and Bruce A. Rideout, D.V.M., Ph.D./ N Engl J Med 2004; 350:1071-1073March 11, 2004

9   Abbas Dehghan, MD, DSC, Mandy van Hoek, MD, Eric J.G. Sijbrands, MD, PHD, Albert Hofman, MD, PhD and Jacqueline C.M. Witteman, PhD. High Serum Uric Acid as a Novel Risk Factor for Type 2 Diabetes Diabetes Care. 2008; 31:361-362

10   Richard J. Johnson, Dan I. Feig, Jaime Herrera-Acosta, Duk-Hee Kang. Resurrection of Uric Acid as a Causal Risk Factor in Essential Hypertension. Hypertension. 2005; 45: 18-20 Published online before print November 22, 2004

policies require that most animals make it to market free of disease. However, there is another "attractive" side effect of antibiotic use: weight gain. Studies have shown that yeast and other fungal extracts given to cattle and pigs cause more intense growth at lower levels of feed intake. Bigger animals, bigger payout, and all this ultimately causes bigger humans. So if the motive of the livestock farmer is money, and more weight means more money, it's a no-brainer why yeast additives form such an integral part of the modern diet of pigs and cattle reared for food. But at what cost? Will we, the consumers, gain weight as a result? Very likely[11].

Yeast is a stressor, because it contains mycotoxins, and these will burn and inflame the body's tissues. Yeast is found in a lot of our foods, and yeast *additives* make foods *addictive*.

Food Pyramid Toxicity

As stated in my first book, *The Hidden Cure*, the introduction of mass-produced leavened bread with its higher levels of rapid rising yeast, together with the overuse of antibiotics such as penicillin and synthetic estrogens, added to a gradual decline in the quality of foods over the last fifty years (medically proven by Doctors McCance and Widdowson) that has caused a massive surge in weight gain, diabetes, high cholesterol, heart disease, and cancer in the boomers.

The McCance and Widdowson report[12] issued the following statement as a conclusion to the effects of the mineral decline in our foods.

---

11   Leveille, Suzanne G., Christina C. Wee, and Lisa I. Iezzoni. "Trends in obesity and arthritis among baby boomers and their predecessors, 1971–2002." *American Journal of Public Health* 95, no. 9 (2005): 1607.

12   A Study on the Mineral Depletion of the Foods Available to us as a Nation over the period 1940–1991. The data used as the basis for this study was published in five editions, initially under the auspices of the Medical Research Council and later the Ministry of Agriculture, Fisheries and Foods, and the Royal Society of Chemistry, authors R. A. McCance and E. M. Widdowson.

That over the last 50 years we have subjected ourselves to an increased environmental toxic load (pesticides, herbicides, fungicides, hormones, heavy metals, antibiotics, colorings, flavorings, preservatives) that is unprecedented in our evolutionary history. Also there has been a radical change in dietary habits towards convenience foods comprised principally of fats, carbohydrates and proteins. As a consequence we have created a society that may be considered overfed yet malnourished of micronutrients. These circumstances contribute significantly towards the rise in chronic disease conditions now present in all age groups – including arthritis, obesity, diabetes, M.S, M.E., osteoporosis, cancer, asthma, eczema, leukemia, cardiovascular diseaseetc.

Could it be wheat allergies[13], with high strains of yeast and antibiotics in the mix, that are giving everybody heart disease and weight gain/diabetes? This might be a cause of dietary stress and inflammation in the gut lining. However, people eat so many grains because they are instructed to by an outdated American food pyramid that recommends six to eleven servings of grain-based foods such as bread (yeast), cereal, noodles, and pastry.

What follows is a diagram of my professional view on what a good food pyramid looks like based on my first book, *The Hidden Cure*. If you compare to a standard food pyramid, it is very different in terms of daily servings of carbohydrates (low GI) and amounts of protein. Excess carbs will feed silent yeast infections that can create stress, hunger, and weight gain.

---

13   Rensch, Michael J., John A. Merenich, Michael Lieberman, Brian D. Long, Dirk R. Davis, and Peter R. McNally. "Gluten-sensitive enteropathy in patients with insulin-dependent diabetes mellitus." Annals of internal medicine 124, no. 6 (1996): 564-567.

```
                    EMF,
                Anti-fungals,
             Vitamins based on pH.

              Xylose Sugar,
             fruits and berries.

       Healthy Fats and oils, such as nuts and seeds,
           salmon oil, flax seeds and olive oil.

       10 -20% Blood type proteins, no more than
    2-3 Oz per meal such as eggs, lamb, chicken, steak,
       turkey, Cornish hens, salmon, red snapper.

   20-30% Low Glycemic index carbohydrates, ground provisions
 such as cassava, pumpkin, squash, yam, dasheen, sweet potato.
    Avoid grains such as wheat flour, oats, gluten grains.

    Plenty of Low Glycemic index vegetables; 60 -80% of the diet should
  be vegetables such as broccoli, zucchini, salads, okra, herbs, tomatoes,
         avocadoes, celery, bok choy, spinach, etc.
```

The Maas Method food pyramid

The Biological Importance of Good Food and our Ancestral Diet

Humans have been eating organic food for thousands upon thousands of years. For as long as time itself, our genetic evolution revolved around the accessibility of good, nourishing food from our clean environment. It's only in the last sixty years that humans have been eating food that has been processed and laced with ever-increasing antibiotic residues, pesticides, and artificial growth hormones. Our children are being born into a very toxic world.

Processed food is making us sick and tired because it does not nourish our bodies to the same degree as organic foods. It's an ancestral issue, because our genes are very fussy about the food quality. They developed in a clean, organic environment, and we should provide them the same today if we want to survive the stress and avoid diseases associated with "modern living." We as a human race have been duped into thinking that fast and processed foods are normal. Our genes are having their say, and stress and weight gain are the response.

Humans need organic energy replacement every three to five hours and material replacement on a daily basis in order to grow and maintain healthy organs. Interestingly, when shedding fat for pre-competition conditioning, bodybuilders will have five, six, or even seven small meals composed entirely of protein, fat, and vegetables. They eat more and lose weight! Crazy, right? However, it's true; it's how bodybuilders shred the fat. Food and timing are key to burning fat and building muscle. The golden rule of bodybuilding is never to feel hungry, because hunger *stalls* the fat-burning properties of the body's hormones. The key here is the type of protein, but more on that later.

When our basic need for food and water is not met, then illness and organ dysfunction will ensue. On an evolutionary level, the operative word is *need*. That need factor is hardwired into our cellular DNA, and as such we look for certain foods today to fulfill that same need. From an osteopathic, homeopathic, and nutritional perspective, our bodies work in harmony only when all our dietary needs are met. That is, when we consume sufficient carbohydrates, proteins, fats, and minerals from our environment, our bodies work well.

When our cells are hungry, they communicate that to our brains through the leptin pathway, and our digestive systems will start to *growl*. Low leptin levels will make us increase our appetite. If this happens, humans will just about eat anything to stop the growl, even if it's junk food. Hunger causes us to search for food and nourishment with *immediacy*. This reflex is as old as the Earth itself. Get food now—search, hunt, look, find, eat. Hunger also makes us emotional, cranky, and snappy as our blood-sugar levels fall. Once the hunger/starving signal has been sent to the brain, the brain then messages via the HPAT axis that the body will store as fat the next food item that is eaten *based on hunger*, in order to have calories saved for a rainy day.

One particular food that makes us hungrier is cheap carbohydrates (e.g. sugar-based items, junk food). The junk-food industry knows that fact about humans too, and its mission statement is to make people eat a food that they love and makes them hungrier for more. They manipulate the food molecules so that people will eat more and more.

Carbohydrates and fats eaten in excess will cause a form of malnutrition that can lead to weight gain, obesity, heart disease, high cholesterol, and diabetes. All these diseases, as papers upon papers of modern research have shown, are linked to the overconsumption of sugars and bad fats, causing us to become ultimately leptin resistant. This is stressful, and being hungry all the time from eating stressful allergic foods creates more stress. The fat trap.

However, if we eat too many cheap trans fats or carbohydrates (laced with antibiotics and fake hormones), our bodies will get sick through the process of leptin resistance, whereby our brains do not respond to leptin and our bodies feel even hungrier. This is happening all over the world right now, spreading as fast as the fast-food restaurant culture as an aspect of modern living.

Our Genes Are Prehistoric, and Our Diet Should Be Too

A hunter-gatherer society[14] is one in which most or all food is obtained from wild plants and animals, in contrast to agricultural societies, which rely mainly on domesticated species. Hunter-gatherers are a type of nomad. Hunting and gathering was the ancestral subsistence mode of mankind. *The Cambridge Encyclopedia*

---

14 F. W. Marlowe, "Hunter-gatherers and human evolution," *Evolutionary Anthropology* 14(2) (2005): 54–67.

of Hunter-Gatherers states that, "Hunting and gathering was humanity's first and most successful adaptation, occupying at least 90 percent of human history. Until 12,000 years ago, all humans lived this way."[15]

In prehistoric times, when food was only obtained through hunting and gathering, we needed to get as much energy from each bite as was humanly possible. Good, high-calorie foods were scarce back in early prehistory. You couldn't get them at the local supermarket, because that concept did not exist. One had to hunt and forage, catch some fish or a deer, and plop it onto the fire, along with wild vegetables and tubers. Life consisted of constantly looking for food. Clearly a very paleo culture.

Following the invention of agriculture, farm culture displaced hunter-gathering groups in most parts of the world. The Neolithic Agricultural Revolution was the world's first historically verifiable revolution in agriculture. It was the broad-scale changeover of many human cultures from a lifestyle of hunting and gathering to one of agriculture and settlement, which supported an increasingly large population[16] and allowed for the development of towns and cities. Archaeological data indicates that the domestication of various forms of plants and animals evolved in separate locations worldwide, starting around twelve thousand years ago[17].

❱ **KEY POINT: Foods packed with higher energy were always in greater demand then (even on a genetic level), because they could save you and your family from starvation. These**

---

15   Richard B. Lee, *Cambridge Encyclopedia of Hunters and Gatherers* (Cambridge: Cambridge University Press, 2005), inside front cover.

16   Jean-Pierre Bocquet-Appel, "When the World's Population Took Off: The Springboard of the Neolithic Demographic Transition," Science 333 (2011): 560–561. Bibcode:2011Sci...333..560B. doi:10.1126/science.1208880. PMID 21798734. Retrieved June 10, 2012.

17   Barker, Graeme. *The Agricultural Revolution in Prehistory: Why did Foragers become Farmers?*: Pg 1-4, Oxford University Press, 2006.

would usually be fat, marrow, honey, and fruits (sugars). However, these precious commodities were always in short supply, and our genes liked them because they were scarce but were very calorie-dense. So we have built into us an old genetic program that yearns for high-energy foods, but that gene program spells disaster for us humans when food is abundant and laced with additives.

Cleaner Paleo Protein and Less Carbs

Early preagricultural people, like cave dwellers, ate a lot more wild organic protein and vegetables, some berries and honey. There is no record of humans knowing how to crystallize sugar in Paleolithic times. The closest things to sugar in nature were honey and fruits. Honey and fruits have vitamins in them; however, sugar that is crystallized is bereft of vitamins through the heating process. Most sugar comes from sugar cane which is a member of the grass family, developed in agricultural times, circa 6000 BC in Papua New Guinea and South East Asia[18].

For early paleo humans, high-calorie foods were stored in the body as fat, and in times of food shortage the fat was broken down into life-giving glucose. Our genes developed a fat-storage system because of these periodic droughts, to ensure we wouldn't starve and die for at least a couple months if we couldn't get adequate nutrition. It would have been the norm that early hunter-gatherer humans would have run out of food periodically.

To safeguard the DNA and reproduction of the species, we evolved a means to *easily* store high-energy foods, such as carbs as fat, for a rainy day so to speak. Credit in the fat bank. However, today we do not readily experience periods of starvation, and as

---

18   Sharpe, Peter. "Sugar cane: past and present." *Ethnobotanical Leaflets* 1998, no. 3 (1998): 6.

such when we eat calorie-dense foods such as sugars, it will easily turn into fat. We instead experience negative emotions and dietary stress as well as chronic pain and inflammation. This sets us up for leptin resistance, whereby the conversion of fat back into sugar slows right down to zero by HFCS, estrogens, and poor food choices and lifestyles, to mention a few causes.

To solve this modern fat/obesity problem, we must learn to eat the way nature designed. Nature created our diets according to our earlier environment, and our genes are still trying to catch up with the shift to modernity. To nudge our bodies in the right direction, we need to consume foods that "reboot" leptin sensitivity and make use of the African mango (Irvingia) and a herbal sugar destroyer (Gymnema) to do just that.

However, we need to get the first fat-burning fuel correct. Our protein choice is critical in burning fat, and that choice is based on our ancestral past.

Paleo-Blood-Type Theory

I will touch upon, and explain the concept of the paleo-blood-type diet now. By studying the images of blood-type distribution across the globe[19], one can start to see a pattern within the data. There must be a link between diet, culture, and environment that shaped the blood-type gene.

Clearly one can see that the greatest density of O bloods are in the Americas, and there are virtually none in Greenland and

---

19   1. Map showing the distribution of the B type blood allele in native populations of the world. reproduced by permission of Oxford University Press. From A. E. Mourant et.al., The Distribution of the Human Blood Groups and Other Polymorphisms, 2nd ed. (1976)
2. Map showing the distribution of the A type blood allele in native populations of the world. Ibid.
3. Map showing the distribution of the O type blood in native populations of the world. Ibid.

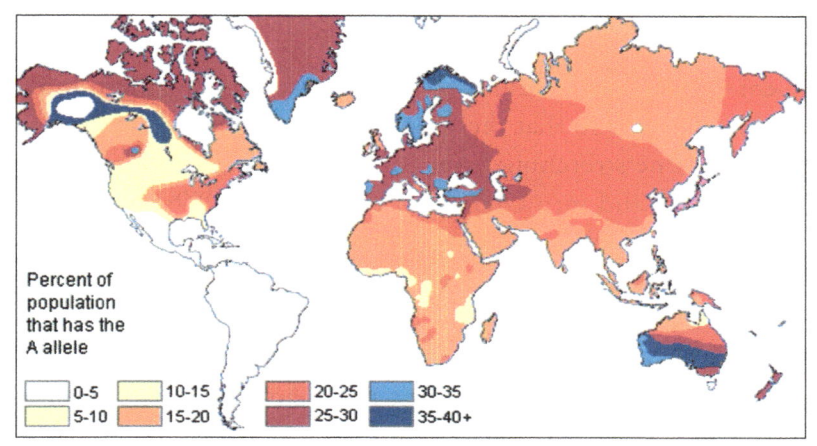

A blood group global distribution

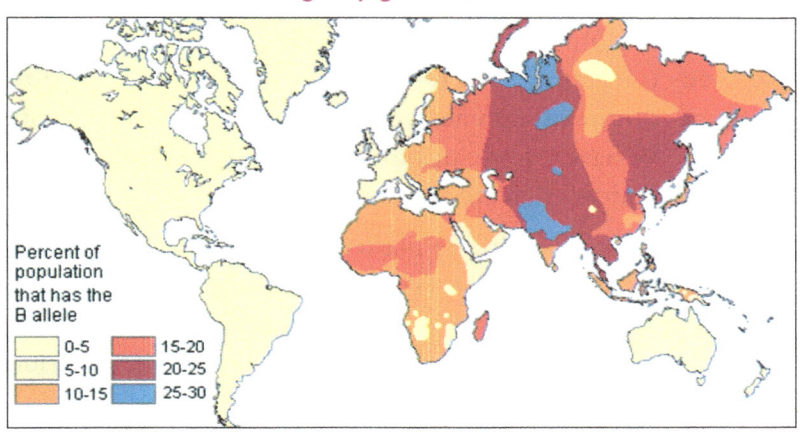

B blood group global distribution.

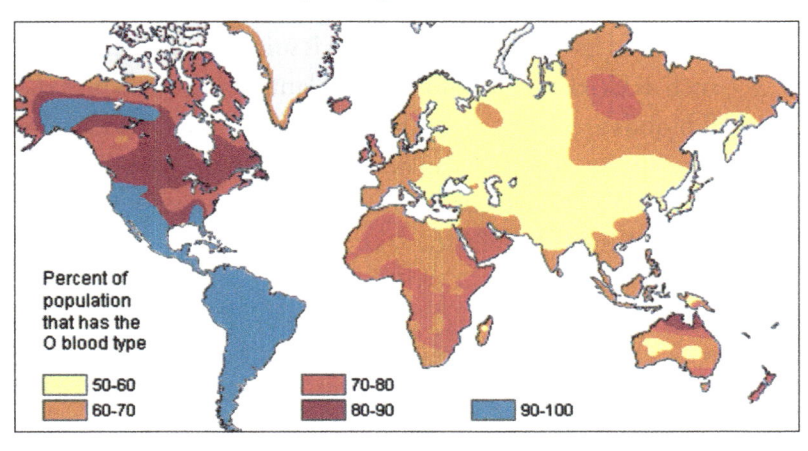

O blood group global distribution.

Central Asia; the B bloods are concentrated in Northern India and Asia; and last, that the A bloods are distributed along the a diagonal line stretching from Australia through to lower Asia and Europe and into Greenland and Canada. What science is telling us now is that when modern humans eat like our paleo ancestors, we benefit from tremendous metabolic and physiological improvements[20].

The key observation here is that different blood groups developed in different environments. Those environments, of course, would have influenced *the culture*, but also, on a deeper level, the environment would have influenced gene function within those blood tribes. Ultimately the way our bodies react to our modern-day foods is nothing short of confused. If we eat according to "our gene" culture environment, our physiology will become more efficient. We have a few clues that we can logically draw from blood-type culture that are as follows:

- O bloods generally are hunter-gatherers (stealth/weapon makers/animal hunters/ foragers), and their digestive systems produced high stomach acid, which is well suited to meat-eating for the primary proteins. Red meat digestion requires more stomach acid.
- A bloods are farmers; they were very aware of time (seed and harvest plants/farm culture) and their digestive systems produced less stomach acid, which is suited to a lighter protein such as chicken, fish and simple plant/grain-based diet.
- B bloods are the nomadic herders and dairy masters, having digestive systems that can handle proteins from lamb, sheep, goat, milk, yogurt, curds, kefirs, and cheeses, yet are allergic to chicken and shellfish.

---

20   Lynda A. Frassetto et al, "Metabolic and physiologic improvements from consuming a paleolithic, hunter-gatherer type diet," *European Journal of Clinical Nutrition* 63.8 (2009): 947–955.

- AB bloods are the moderns (city dwellers/traders/silk road merchants); they have the best and the worst features of the A and B blood types.

This is only a simplistic guide, but it seems to be effective in my clinical practice. However, some people have allergy issues that need to be individually tested to figure out more about specific allergies that they silently have to foods, beverages, herbs and spices.

Later in the book, in the chapter called "Creating Your Fat-Burning Plate," I will describe to you what your paleo-blood-type diet should be, which includes an important piece about metabolic-type diet and figuring how much carbs you can have per day, versus protein. However, our environment and the low quality of proteins that represent it has changed for the worse. Modern Frankenfoods are being produced en masse with the general masses not realizing that most of the food they eat daily is fake. Choose carefully; your future body shape depends on your wise choice.

Chapter 2

Chemicals, Antibiotics, Yeast, and Fungus Are Stressful

Penicillin, the best-selling and most internationally known drug, is actually a fungal-based medicine prescribed as an antibiotic. Penicillin the drug is a purified mycotoxin from the fungus *Penicillium chrysogenum*. In the 1990s US doctors prescribed approximately 200–250 million antibiotic prescriptions to their patients.

While the use of penicillin and other antibiotics has been an important step in improving the health and life span of the human race, it is not without its negative consequences. Other penicillin species are used to make the mold of Brie, Camembert, Gorgonzola, and Danish blue cheeses. The overuse of antibiotics in commercial farming has gained benefits to the farmer, but it has created antibiotic-resistant species of bacteria[1].

Cancer has its roots in fungus, so it should be no surprise that fungal-based medicines can cause cancer. As we have already discussed, they destroy friendly bacteria and irritate human cells by setting up a fungal allergy stress response. It is now accepted among the scientific community that penicillin can cause lymphoma in humans[2]. If a drug can induce a disease, then the body must view the drug as a stressor. Mineral depletion can be a cause of the

---

1 Nichole Johnston, "Farming Antibiotic Threat: The use of drugs to make animals grow larger has led to the emergence of antibiotic-resistant bacteria in the food chain," *Globe and Mail*, September 26 Archives.foodsafety.ksu.edu, Guelph University, Canada 2000.

2 Prof. A V Costantini et Al, Breast cancer, Hope At Last Fungalbionic series of books; WHO Collaborating Centre for Mycotoxins in Foods, (J Verlag publishing, Germany1998) Chp 9 pg 40

stress, or it could be the loss of normal microflora in the gut. Dr. Pelton, a pharmacist in the US, lists the major nutrients that are depleted as a consequence of antibiotic therapy as follows[3]:

- Bifidobacteria (friendly bacteria)
- Biotin
- Inositol
- Lactobacillus acidophilus (friendly bacteria)
- Vitamin B1, B2, B3, B6, B12
- Vitamin K

The WHO's Professor Costantini, MD, clearly showed the links to these diseases in his exhaustive research for the *Fungalbionic* book series[4], which medically describes the links between breast cancer, prostate cancer, heart disease, and high blood pressure, and discusses how they are all somehow related to human fungal exposure through the consumption of foods and medications that carry fungal spores and mycotoxins. As I wrote in *The Hidden Cure*:

> Fungi and yeasts grow by fermentation and the byproducts of their metabolism, such as lactic acid, carbon dioxide, alcohol, and acetaldehydes; all these can pickle the liver and irritate the pancreas. Unfortunately, the cells of the liver and pancreas will eventually come to a point where the toxic deluge can overwhelm ordinary cell function and damage the organs. Yeasts can also produce large amounts of uric acid, which in turn can induce diabetes, arthritis, kidney disease, heart disease, and leukemia. Uric acid is a toxic metabolite of yeasts and fungi. Professor Costantini is of the opinion, backed by thorough research, that the high uric acid levels found in the blood of gout and diabetic

---

3 Ross Pelton RPh, PhD et al, *Drug Induced Nutrient Depletion handbook*, (Lexi-Comp Clinical Reference Library, Canada 1999-2000) Pg. 76

4 A. V. Costantini, H. Wieland, and L. I. Qvick, Fungalbionic Series: *Atherosclerosis, Hope at Last*, World Health Organization Collaborating Centre for Mycotoxins in Foods Freiburg, Germany: Johann Friedrich Oberlin Verlag Publishers, 1998

patients is likely of fungal origin. This key insight explains why I see so many diabetic patients who also have serious arthritic, heart, and kidney disease.

Yeast and fungus have the capability of producing many mycotoxins, one of which is uric acid. High levels of uric acid have been linked to leukemia and kidney disease[5].

This yeast/fungal connection explains why extremely low-GI diets, such as the Atkins or South Beach Diet, work to reduce cholesterol and heart disease because both of these are linked to yeast overgrowth. Long-term, however, there is a high dropout rate for the Atkins Diet simply because you just can't starve yourself of all carbs for a sustained period of time.

My dietary approach to sugar replacement is and sweetener called xylitol or xylose, which is completely natural. The human body produces small amounts of xylose daily, approximately 15–20mg. Xylose is exclusively processed by the liver and *not* the pancreas, hence the benefits of this sugar for diabetics. Bodybuilders use xylose sugar with great success, shedding body fat to show rippling muscles.

Xylose sugar will not feed yeast or fungus or even a bacterium. Xylose requires *no insulin* for its management because the GI is so low!

It has a 5-carbon sugar, which makes it very special in that microbes and fungi can only metabolize a 6-carbon sugar and not a 5-carbon sugar molecule. This way the body and brain get fed their caloric need for sugars without the fat deposition and the promotion of microbes within the body. Xylose is good for patients with diabetes, as it only has a glycemic index of 7! Those sensitive to xylitol could use erythritol instead.

---

[5] Richard E. Rieselbach et al, "Uric acid excretion and renal function in the acute hyperuricemia of leukemia: pathogenesis and therapy of uric acid nephropathy," *The American Journal of Medicine* 37.6 (1964): 872–884.

Obesogens: A New Suspect in Metabolic Disruption

America's weight problems may be from more than just eating too much and exercising too little. Researchers are putting forward the theory that obesogens, otherwise known as endocrine disrupting chemicals (EDCs), are a major cause of ill health and disease. EDCs are chemicals known to cause dysfunction within hormonal systems and cause imbalance in homeostasis. These are a class of natural and synthetic compounds thought to cause anything from obesity and cancer to heart disease and diabetes.

Bruce Blumberg, PhD, School of Biological Sciences of the University of California, Irvine, has researched the link between obesity, fungicides, and pesticides[6]. He coined the term *obesogens*. Blumberg's groundbreaking work effectively showed that pesticides and pollution played a role in the causation of obesity in young lab rats and the rat model evidence could comfortably explain the high occurrence of obesity even in very young babies and toddlers.

The problem goes even further than the overweight individual or family, in that epigenetic studies have shown that children of future generations can suffer from the same diseases. Recently an article published by the BBC World News titled "Obesity 'often set before the age of two,'" described how researchers in the US found in a study of more than one hundred obese children and teenagers that more than 90 percent of them were overweight by the age of five, and 25 percent of them were overweight by just five months old[7]!

---

6   Felix Grün and Bruce Blumberg, "Endocrine disrupters as Obesogens," *Molecular and Cellular Endocrinology* 304(1–2) (2009) 19–29. (http://www.sciencedirect.com/science/article/pii/S0303720709001488)

7   http://news.bbc.co.uk/2/hi/health/8512102.stm?Obesity-'set'-before-age-of-two

Exposure to environmental chemicals during pregnancy[8] may be a factor in the obesity epidemic currently seen today, as more children are diagnosed with obesity at earlier ages. There are young children who already suffer from high cholesterol. Remember the days when high cholesterol was only regarded as an aging disease?

The sources of these EDCs or obesogens can be meat tainted with synthetic hormones and yeast additives, some plastics, pesticides, DDT, dioxins, industrial chemicals, pollution, or pharmaceutical agents. Even natural chemicals such as genistein from soy, a type of phytoestrogen, can cause havoc to the endocrine system in some cases of abnormal genetic liver metabolism.

Obesogens are thought to create havoc with the regulation of hormones within the body, probably switching on more *estrogenic functions* and contributing to the lowering of testosterone, therefore contributing to weight gain. The endocrine system of the body is finely tuned using a feedback system. EDCs or obesogens cause the body's glandular systems to stay switched on too long.

Strange chemicals become unnaturally implanted on the receptor sites of various glands, such as the thyroid or pancreas, causing the gland either to slow down or speed up. This can be seen clearly due to the bee populations going into rapid decline. The bees are our environmental marker as to the state of the natural systems, and as they are in serious decline[9] and could potentially collapse the food chain[10], is it any great stretch of the imagination

---

[8] Bucala, Richard, Jack Fishman, and Anthony Cerami. "Formation of covalent adducts between cortisol and 16 alpha-hydroxyestrone and protein: possible role in the pathogenesis of cortisol toxicity and systemic lupus erythematosus." *Proceedings of the National Academy of Sciences* 79, no. 10 (1982): 3320-3324.

[9] Mickaël Henry, Maxime Béguin, Fabrice Requier, Orianne Rollin, Jean-François Odoux, Pierrick Aupinel, Jean Aptel, Sylvie Tchamitchian, and Axel Decourtye, "A Common Pesticide Decreases Foraging Success and Survival in Honey Bees ," *Science* 20 (2012): 348–350.Published online 29 March 2012.

[10] Erik Stokstad, "Field Research on Bees Raises Concern About Low-Dose Pesticides," *Science* 30 (2012): 1555.

to conclude that pesticides are damaging so many creatures[11], including humans?

The Progressive Estrogenization of our Environment

Over the decades, synthetic estrogens (which are made from petrochemicals) have taken their toll on the health of the Earth's entire population. It is a by-product of the industrialization that has occurred since World War II. Estrogen and antibiotic residues are evident in our widely accepted food pyramid and supply chain. Those who unknowingly consume these foods actually set themselves up for weight gain, diabetes, and worse still, cancer[12] or heart disease[13],[14].

The problems with weight gain are not purely aesthetic. Directly proportional to an increase in weight is an elevated risk of diabetes, heart disease, and death. The roots of our major illnesses are fungus and yeast, pesticides, synthetic hormones, xenobiotics, bad fat and oils, xenoestrogens, and obesogens[15]. These ingredients, *when combined* with a decrease in the hormones that burn fat (like progesterone, DHEA, and testosterone) and an

---

11 Rozen, Daniel E. "Drugged bees go missing." The Journal of Experimental Biology 215, no. 17 (2012): iv-iv.-http://jeb.biologists.org/content/215/17/iv.short

12 Dany Chalbos, Francoise Vignon, Iafa Keydar, and Henri Rochefort, "Estrogens Stimulate Cell Proliferation and Induce Secretory Proteins in a Human Breast Cancer Cell Line (T47D)," JCEM 55 (1982): 276–283.

13 Katerina Saltiki and Maria Alevizaki. "Coronary heart disease in postmenopausal women; the role of endogenous Estrogens and their receptors," *Hormones* 6(1) (2007): 9–24.

14 Women's health: Preventing the top 7 threats, http://www.mayoclinic.com/health/wom-ens-health/WO00014

15 Evanthia Diamanti-Kandarakis, Jean-Pierre Bourguignon, Linda C. Giudice, Russ Hauser, Gail S. Prins, Ana M. Soto, R. Thomas Zoeller, and Andrea C. Gore. "Endocrine-Disrupting Chemicals: An Endocrine Society Scientific Statement," *Endocrine Reviews* 30(4) (2009): 293–342.

increase in the hormones that store fat (insulin, estrogen, and cortisol) can result in a deadly recipe for obesity and ill health.

Despite today's hustling, bustling, hyper-estrogenized environment, our genes are still stuck in this "carb to fat" storage mode, even if we follow a regular meal system of fat, simple sugars, and carbs at breakfast, lunch, and dinner. Leptin resistance ensues, and the weight piles on as appetite and stress increase during life.

Now do you see what you have to deal with in order to burn fat? Estrogen actually *stimulates* the fat cells to grow, making you want to eat more and more food.

Pesticides Disrupt Our Hormone Balance

Pesticides are known to cause thyroid dysfunctions, and DDT and DDE, like the killer pesticides from the 1960s, can cause obesity, breast cancer, and endometriosis.

Foods wrapped in plastic carry a compound called bisphenol A (BPA) that permeates the food, creating an estrogen-like effect and thereby aiding in the feminization of men and overfeminization of women. Let me remind you here that testosterone creates muscular bodies and estrogen creates flabby bodies. BPA is linked to infant obesity in the rat model[16].

Even though the public was formerly being misled about the dangers of BPA, many supermarket shelves continue to use this estrogen-based plastic[17], thereby spreading the disease of weight gain and obesity.

---

16   H. Masuno, T. Kidani, K. Sekiya, K. Sakayama, T. Shiosaka, H. Yamamoto, et al, "Bisphenol A in combination with Insulin can accelerate the conversion of 3T3-L1 fibroblasts to adipocytes," *Journal of Lipid Researchs*. 43(5) (2002):676–684.

17   F. S. vom Saal, S. C. Nagel, B. G. Timms, and W. V. Welshons, "Implications for human health of the extensive bisphenol A literature showing adverse effects at low doses: a response to attempts to mislead the public," *Toxicology* 212(2–3) (2005): 244–252.

The concept that obesity is caused by environmental issues and EDCs is gaining greater understanding. The chemicals and hormones (obesogens) we have put into the environment are now coming back through the food chain and slowly making people fat, susceptible to lifestyle disease, and potentially killing everybody. Obesogens foster yeast infections, as the body's metabolism remains out of homeostasis and becomes overly acidic and estrogenic.

Water and Toothpaste Is Making Me Fat?

Fluoridation of water, endorsed by the US government, has also been heavily scrutinized by the current Environmental Protection Agency (EPA) and is now deemed to be a health hazard[18] with research stating that fluoride may be in part responsible for the obesity epidemic facing America[19]. This is a quote from the fluoride research article.

> The epidemic of obesity is worldwide. It will be followed by an epidemic of diabetes. Although there is a genetic basis for obesity and diabetes, the current epidemic reflects the failure of our ancient genes to cope with a modern toxic environment. To put it another way, the genetic background loads the gun, but the environment pulls the trigger. Diet, lifestyle and exercise are the cornerstones of current approaches to treating obesity.

In an interview, Dr. Richard Shames, a renowned physician dealing with thyroid disorders, drew attention to a statement that ought to be of particular interest. The statement—from the employees union of the Environmental Protection Agency—was

---

18   http://thyroid.about.com/cs/toxicchemicalsan/a/flouride.htm
19   G. A. Bray, Hypothesis. Pennington Biomedical Research Center, "The epidemic of obesity and changes in food intake: the Fluoride Hypothesis" Physiology & Behavior, Volume 82, Issue 1, August 2004, Pages 115–121, *Europe Pub Med Central* (2004) http://ukpmc.ac.uk/abstract/MED/15234599-

released on January 2, 1997, and represented fifteen hundred scientists, engineers, lawyers, and other professionals at EPA headquarters in Washington, DC. It reads:

> Our members' review of the body of evidence over the last 11 years, including animal and human epidemiology studies, indicates a causal link between fluoride/fluoridation and cancer, genetic damage, neurological impairment, and bone pathology.
>
> ...Our research of older medical articles revealed that fluoride was once used as an anti-thyroid medicine, prescribed by doctors in hospitals and clinics. It was used to slow down an overactive thyroid. In addition, it was also effective in slowing down a normal or already-sluggish hypothyroid gland. For instance, in the *Journal of Clinical Endocrinology*, Volume 18, 1958, page 1102, Drs. Galetti and Goyer explain the "Effect of Fluorine in Thyroidal Iodine Metabolism in Hyperthyroidism."

So fluoride appears to reduce the activity of the thyroid gland, and in turn your metabolism slows down and you could gain weight. The thyroid gland plays a very important role in the health of human metabolism, and clearly there are many modern chemicals, such as fluoride, that can cause it to become disrupted and induce hypothyroidism, cancer, or autoimmune diseases.

Dr. Shames has also stated, "We now feel convinced that the thyroid epidemic could be due largely to the excessive harmful chemicals in our food, air, and water, confusing and stressing our immune systems."

Even fluoride toothpaste, hailed as a preventer of tooth decay for decades, is now regarded as a competitive thyroid disruptor. Fluorine is a cousin to iodine, which is also a member of the halogen family. Iodine is essential for normal thyroid function, and fluoride will compete with the docking sites of the thyroid gland, inducing a hypothyroidism. Conclusion : Even using the wrong toothpaste can cause you to put on weight

So hold on. Let's get this straight. Over the last fifty years, sugar has been packed into people's meals; the land has been laced with petrochemicals (xenoestrogens), antibiotics, and yeast residues; synthetic growth hormones have been given left, right, and center; the atmosphere has been intoxicated; and to crown it all off, consumers have been convinced that brushing with sodium fluoride toothpaste (a pesticide) will protect their teeth. (If that's true, then why is there a poison-control statement on every tube of toothpaste that contains sodium fluoride?)

At least some people will die (twenty-five to thirty years earlier, from heart disease, cancer, diabetic complications, and obesity with poor quality of health) with a shiny smile, thanks to fluoride-based toothpaste.

The general misunderstanding about people gaining weight is that it is *not* that they "couldn't stick to a diet" or that they couldn't burn fat because "they're a loser"...it's really a matter of a toxic environment, addiction to sugar and yeast, and hormone havoc. The dice are loaded and the deck is stacked, dooming most weight loss diets to failure.

All this excessive stress creates a massive chemical imbalance. Overweight people eat too much and store it as fat because of chemicals and hormones that have become imbalanced because they are programmed to do that in farm animals.

Our environment can make an unsuspecting human become gluttonous; that's how the food companies get people to eat more of their foods.

❯ **KEY POINT: Let's get real about this basic point: eat lots of sugars and carbohydrates, and your body will make lots of a fat-storage hormone called insulin. If you eat pesticide-laced food and use fluoride-based toothpaste, it will disrupt the balance of the eight hormones that control your weight, mood, and sleep function.**

Too much insulin in the blood means that you cannot burn fat; the insulin signal within the body says build more fat cells.

Lower insulin equals better fat burn. If you get your insulin and blood sugars level, you will burn fat. Get your blood sugar to stay within 80–100mg/dl. Look at the glycemic chart. See if you can float within that fat-burn zone. Following is a diagram of how insulin responds to sugars and carbs. The fat-burn zone is shown to be balanced in the middle between 80–100mg/dl.

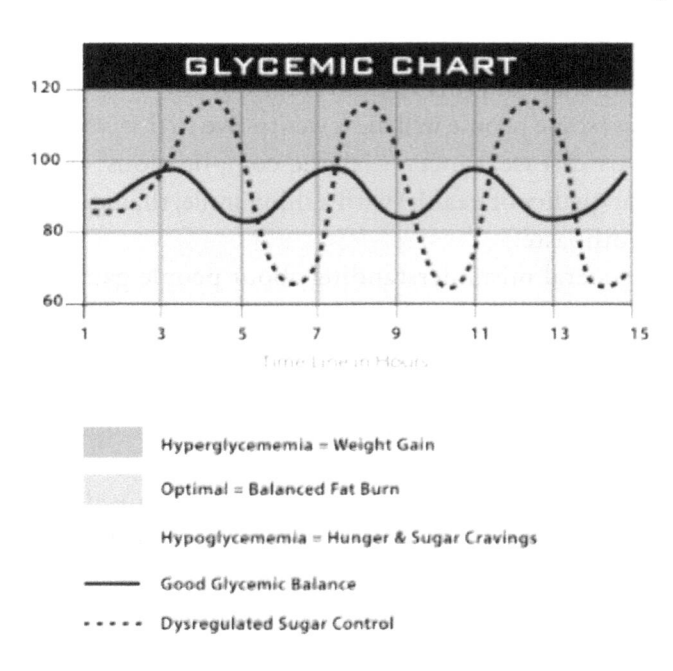

GLYCEMIC CHART

Hyperglycememia = Weight Gain

Optimal = Balanced Fat Burn

Hypoglycememia = Hunger & Sugar Cravings

—— Good Glycemic Balance

· · · · · Dysregulated Sugar Control

Glycemic chart.

If you want to lose weight and burn fat, you have to keep your sugars steady by trying to keep the levels between 80–100mg/dl. It's the only scientific way. Keep the sugars in the blood under good control, and you will stop building fat cells—especially around the stomach!

Jorge Cruise has explored this quite well in *The Belly Fat Cure*. As we will soon find out, serious weight loss is not just about carb control; as you now understand, it involves correcting our stress levels and our hormone balance, and it's also about the **bad**

estrogens and high levels of **cortisol** that throw off the thyroid balance and sleep cycle that can cause us to be fat.

So sugars and carbohydrates are only one fraction in the Total Fat Cure equation. However, another component of this quandary is hormones, particularly how to lower the levels of the fat-causing hormone estrogen and boost the levels of the fat-burning hormone testosterone. Estrogen will give an individual a classic apple body shape. Have you ever noticed that many overweight people have that typical body shape?

Clues from the Bodybuilders

However, another subsection of the population—bodybuilders—have identical body shapes, but in the opposite situation. Line them off on a stage, and you will see that all of them have the same well-developed muscularity. How did they get there?

❱ **KEY POINT: They achieve this by boosting their testosterone levels and *lowering* estrogen within their bodies.**

If you want an athletic body, it really comes down to the hormones coursing through your veins and how they relate to your diet and environment. It's that simple. This is one of the key clue *antidotes* to the obesity epidemic. Build muscle to help burn fat. Testosterone is a fat burner and a muscle-building hormone. You can't get a muscle to burn fat and rebuild stronger unless there are adequate levels of testosterone.

Bodybuilders have taught us one of the most important ways of transforming our bodies into fantastic fat blasters. When it comes to the perfect physique, bodybuilders are a class apart. Their physical and mental discipline is admirable, and their vanity expressed in achieving excellence is unparalleled. They have used their vanity to overcome the daunting obstacle of fat metabolism. They have paved the way in shredding fat by using some very cool techniques.

They avoid starchy carbs entirely because starch and sugar cause the body to hold on to its fat reserves. They ramp up their testosterone levels (naturally or synthetically) and put the brakes on their estrogens so that they burn incredible amounts of fat. They clearly know how to derail our human metabolic train track from carb burn to fat burn. Bodybuilders will only use carbohydrates and starches when they want to bulk up weight. Some favorites seem to be yams and sweet potatoes, as they are low in the glycemic index. When shredding, fat they always have a piece of protein in their stomachs in between meals to switch off the hunger signal.

Now, you don't have to be a bodybuilder to achieve body perfection, you just have to model their techniques and be disciplined enough to *avoid eating excess carbs*, by reducing your stress and switching off the hunger signal, by using proteins very carefully.

Don't be afraid to be a little tough on yourself. The plain fact is that there's twice as much energy in fat than in carbs. You have got to get back into a better energy-production system in order to lose weight, and proteins are at the core because they help stabilize sugar and promote fat burning.

> **KEY POINT: Our bodies are designed to eat more protein and fat as well as vegetable-based minerals to survive. Back in Paleolithic times, only a small fraction of the caloric intake would have been from sugars and starch. Our bodies function much better with a low-carb diet. Carbs carry a lot of energy, and storing this energy over time causes fat. Insulin turns sugar into fat. Protein creates a better metabolism and fat burn and helps to balance insulin and activate our thyroids.**

Lifestyle Check

Each year thousands of patients consult with me via Skype/ telephone / physically from all over the world to achieve their health goals. Whether they want to recover from an illness or a disease, or just lose weight and feel better, the starting point is always the same: creating a long-term **plan** to be healthy for the rest of their lives. Using this book you can create a new lifestyle for yourself that self-heals.

This is a lifestyle program, and anything less than that will fail. By becoming healthy, you are creating a new lifestyle and vice versa. Talk to anyone who is slim and fit and they will most likely tell you that their secret is eating right and exercising regularly (two or three times per week). They also possess good hormone balance.

That's just the start. You also have to think positively in order to do all the things you need to do to make your new life happen and get results. Discipline to eat well and exercise the muscles regularly breeds success, but get your hormones balanced.

❱ **KEY POINT: Muscles are metabolically very active, and we use the energy burnt from our fats and sugars to make our muscles more active. Extra muscle will burn more fat. Fat, on the other hand, is metabolically inactive. Overtraining will hurt muscles and cause them to break down, whereas undertraining will cause them to go flabby. If we want to become slim, we have to enhance our muscle growth with the right amount of stimulus to do just that. Muscles help you to lose weight, so exercise is vital to keeping the fat off as well as helping the body stay young. See the chapter "Strong Body."**

Everyone Can Burn Fat. It's Hardwired into Our DNA.

We're genetically equipped with the ability to burn fat. We all can produce the key hormones called leptin and adiponectin, and these are the body's key fat-burning hormones used in conjunction with the adrenal hormones, thyroid and sex hormones. More on this later. However, there is a very small percentage of humans who have "genetic obesity," states Dr. Joseph Majzoub[20],

---

20   Alexandra Sifferlin, "New Genes ID'd in Obesity: How Much of Weight is Genetic?" *Time* July 16, 2013http://healthland.time.com/2013/07/19/news-genes-idd-in-obesity-how-much-of-weight-is-genetic

chief MD of the Endocrine division of Boston Children's Hospital.

> Thus far mutations in about eight genes are known to cause obesity in humans. But these mutations account for under five percent of the obesity in our society, and certainly are not, by themselves, responsible for the current obesity epidemic, since the mutation rate in these genes could not have changed dramatically during the past twenty years," says Dr. Joseph Majzoub, the chief of the division of endocrinology at Boston Children's Hospital and an author on the Science paper. "However, mutations in these genes have led to the discovery of pathways that are important in energy balance in humans, giving us hope that drugs can be developed that affect these pathways to prevent excessive weight gain, either by curbing appetite or increased burning of calories.

So for those of us who have extra weight piling on, for most it can't be genetic and has to be environmental issues that are switching some fat-gain switch. When we get stressed, we pile on the weight, especially around the middle belly area, the cortisol belly.

Leptin and adiponectin hormones are *genetically wired* to help your body fat be a reserve of stored energy, a sort of stress fat bank that was really important when food was scarce back in ancestral times. Having high levels of leptin/adiponectin is key in the fat-burning process. If you were to starve, the body's leptin/adiponectin levels would drop, thereby decreasing the rate at which fat is burnt, self-protectively causing hunger and the search for food.

These days people try to lose weight but can't because they are fighting a genetic hormone program that protects you from starvation. Most fat people these days are leptin resistant and have low levels of adiponectin, so they are hungry most of the time. Some of my patients sleepwalk to the fridge and eat large amounts of cheap calories at night. Fat and obese people have high levels of leptin, but the leptin is bounded to a blood protein CRP

(C-reactive protein) that renders it ineffective. Fat people have low levels of adiponectin because of the leptin resistance. There is a domino effect from stress.

All we have to do is create the right circumstances for fat burning to be efficient. We know scientifically that you can get energy not only from sugars and carbs, but also from good fats, proteins, and vegetables, but also *you can get calories from burning your own fats.*

The keys here are leptin/adiponectin. If you want to burn fat you'll need to learn about leptin and adiponectin and how they relate. Leptin and adiponectin resistance comes about from a diet of high sugars and processed foods. The trick is, how do you repair the pathway to switch on the fat burn? You will find out a scientific and natural way to do just that shortly.

Fact: fat gives you double the energy of carbohydrates, but you have to be able to make a metabolic switch from a practiced carb burner to a born-again fat burner. Making that leptin switch is what this book is about. There's a crucial point when people who switch from carb burning to fat burning have to be disciplined for about two or three days for the handover to take place. Bodybuilders know this carb withdrawal very well, and as they cut carbs to define muscle, their bodies have no choice but to change into fat-burner mode. However, bodybuilders know that there is an African mango extract and an old ayurvedic herb that allows them to restore leptin sensitivity and keep the appetite low, balancing their blood sugars, that keeps hunger away and keeps them burning fats at a higher rate together with a fantastic protein/fat/veggie carb diet.

If you burn fat, you will reverse numerous lifestyle diseases quite quickly at the same time, because your body was designed to eat carbs and sugars only in very small amounts and to eat proteins and vegetables in large amounts. High carbs create disease.

Before we launch into the Total Fat Cure, we must understand why we eat and how our evolution shaped the way we live in our environment. We all know that a high-carb, high-fat diet is dangerous to our health, as it damages the leptin and adiponectin pathways that help us to maintain our body-fat percentage at a healthy level.

However, we are instinctively hardwired to choose these high-carb foods because they contain a lot of energy. But why are we so thirsty for this energy?

Evolution. Our prehistoric environment didn't have carb calorie–dense foods, so when we ate those foods, our bodies would save the energy as fat for a rainy day when food was not so plentiful. One of the biggest stressors in prehistory was when humans ran out of food. Starvation was a very real threat to the well-being of the tribe. If humans starved a little, their bodies would go into emergency fat-storage mode with the next meal. Hence delaying or skipping meals causes us to gain weight through the starvation response. However, if there is some protein in the stomach, the hunger switches off and the metabolism continues.

Locusts Can Help Our Understanding of Obesity

Locusts have huge appetites, and they literally are one of the greatest pests in the world, second only to mosquitoes. They attack huge tracts of crops and cause massive devastation. They move in the thousands, like armies swarming, devouring everything green in their path just to get their greedy fill of plant-based proteins.

Swarms can eat tens of thousands of tons of vegetable matter. The Americas, Australia, Asia, and Africa all suffer the effects of locusts.

Plant proteins are essential to us because our genes (DNA) are made from proteins, and the only way a locust can reproduce is with protein. So their survival, like many other creatures, depends on their ability to correctly feed and reproduce.

Professor Stephen Simpson of the School of Biological Sciences at Sydney University[21] has discovered something very interesting

21 http://www.unileverhealthcarenutrition.com.au/Files/Perspectives/Perspectives

about locusts and crickets[22]. He has understood what controls their appetite to feed and to become obese[23].

Locusts will continue to eat more carbs until they are satisfied that they have gained enough *protein from within* those carbs. Protein-rich diets create thinner, more agile locusts that fly better, and of course they survive danger and predation far greater than a fatter locust.

If locusts have a high-carb, low-protein diet, they get fat and likelier to be eaten.

> **KEY POINT:** In our high carb–laden society, people will continue eating carbs and more carbs until they have managed to get the right amount of protein from that chosen carb. Many snacks are just pure sugar carbs that raise insulin, which swings the body into fat-storage mode. This is a diet-based stress response. We need to eat correct amounts and types of protein with some carbs in the right ratio.

%20-%20May%202009.pdf

22   S. J. Simpson, G. A. Sword, P. D. Lorch, and I. D. Couzin, "Cannibal crickets on a forced march for protein and salt," Proc Natl Acad Sci U S A. 103(11) (2006): 4152–4156. Epub 2006 Mar 3 *School of Biological Sciences*, University of Sydney, Heydon-Laurence Building A08, Sydney NSW 2006

23   http://sydney.edu.au/about/profile/our_people/power_of_protein.shtml

Chapter 3

Weight Gain and the Eight Fat Hormones

In the process of losing weight by burning fat, you will want to become familiar with the eight key hormones that control the way you look in terms of how much fat your body will retain.

1. Cortisol—Stress defines the biological reaction of your body to an emotional pressure, physical threat, or spiritual fear. It manifests itself as a surge in adrenal-gland function. Over time these "stress" surges result in an overall decline in adrenal hormone production. Cortisol is a glucocorticosteroid, so every time cortisol rises, so do sugar levels in the blood. Chronic anxiety, constant worry, nervous tension, work pressure, hassle, inability to relax, sleep deprivation, allergies, parasites, physical trauma, and more will raise cortisol and adrenaline, and over time that will wear the body and its organs down into disease. Cortisol is catabolic so it breaks down tissue.

2. Insulin—Ancient Egyptian and Grecian physicians were aware of diabetes, but they didn't recognize its relation to a diseased pancreas. The Greek physician Aretaeus coined the term *diabetes* in the first century AD. It means "siphon" due to the symptom of fluid loss from excessive urination. Early physicians could not treat diabetes, and so their patients slowly wasted away. Diabetes today is one of the fastest-growing epidemics in the world and is responsible for killing approximately 5 percent of the

world's population[1]. Balancing carbs and proteins is key to recovery[2].

3. **Estrogens**—Synthetic estrogens have been in our environment since their mass introduction into society post–World War II. Birth control, hormone-replacement therapy, plastics, and cosmetics are all made up of estrogen-like molecules. For most people, a gradual estrogen effect manifests itself in the form of degenerative disease[3]. Women take estrogen in hormone-replacement therapy and birth-control pills. Our diets and even common household products are laced with estrogen[4]. Men with excess estrogen become fat[5], have male boobs, prostate disorders[6], and diabetes[7].

---

1   Emma Farnsworth, Natalie D. Luscombe, Manny Noakes, Gary Wittert, Eleni Argyiou, and Peter M Clifton. "Effect of a high-protein, energy-restricted diet on body composition, Glycemic control, and lipid concentrations in overweight and obese hyperInsulinemic men and women," *American Journal of Clinical Nutrition* 78(1) (2003): 31–39.

2   N. H. Baba, S. Sawaya, N. Torbay, Z. Habbal, S. Azar, and S. A. Hashim, "High protein vs. high carbohydrate hypoenergetic diet for the treatment of obese hyperInsulinemic subjects," *Journal of the International Association for the Study of Obesity* 23(11) (1999):1202–1206.

3   Wood CE et Al, Effects of Estradiol with micronized progesterone or medroxyprogesterone acetate on risk markers for breast cancer in postmenopausal monkeys, Breast Cancer Research Treat; 101:125–134. *US National Library of Medicine National Institutes of Health* 2007

4   Dany Chalbos, Francoise Vignon, Iafa Keydar, and Henri Rochefort, "Estrogens Stimulate Cell Proliferation and Induce Secretory Proteins in a Human Breast Cancer Cell Line (T47D)," *JCEM* 55 (1982): 276–283.

5   SCHNEIDER, GEORGE, MARVIN A. KIRSCHNER, RICHARD BERKOWITZ, and NORMAN H. ERTEL. "Increased Estrogen Production in Obese Men*." *The Journal of Clinical Endocrinology & Metabolism* 48, no. 4 (1979): 633-638.

6   Ulrich Seppelt, "Correlation among Prostate Stroma, Plasma Estrogen Levels, and Urinary Estrogen Excretion in Patients with Benign Prostatic Hypertrophy," *JCEM* 47 (1978): 1230–1235.

7   L. Maas, BSc, Ost, DIHom, Curing Diabetes in Seven Steps (*Wheatmark Press*, AZ: 2012), p.80.

4. **Thyroid**—This gland situated in the front of the neck is associated with energy and metabolism. As the levels of thyroid hormones drop over time due to stress, chronic use of fluoride-based toothpaste, allergies, and low DHEA and progesterone levels, your metabolic rate slows down. The thyroid is easily affected by environmental chemicals such as fluoride (found in toothpaste), bromine (found in baked goods), and chlorine (found in drinking water). Hypothyroidism is pandemic around the world, and is it any wonder, as most humans use fluoride-based toothpaste and eat baked goods?

5. **Leptin**—This is a key hormone that deals with energy and appetite. Lowering the carbs too much and for too long can lower your leptin levels, and this will slow your fat metabolism and increase appetite. Having a small amount of carbs keeps the leptin levels normal and maintains fat metabolism. The absence of leptin causes uncontrolled food ingestion that can cause obesity. Mild weight gain can eventually lead to leptin resistance. Improve your leptin levels by avoiding high-fructose corn syrup (HFCS), as this sugar can cause leptin resistance.

6. **Adiponectin**—This hormone is produced from fat tissue itself, and just like leptin, adiponectin will cause an increase in fat metabolism. Both leptin and adiponectin are closely related to each other in function. Recent research has uncovered that adiponectin is directly related to obesity and the development of T2 diabetes. This hormone protein regulates insulin sensitivity in humans, and the general rule is that the more fat the person is carrying, the lower the adiponectin levels in their blood. By increasing adiponectin levels, weight loss is created and the risk of diabetes reduces. Diet and exercise will encourage a rise

in adiponectin[8]. Increasing your fish oils and magnesium levels through supplements and five servings of vegetables daily can also increase adiponectin.

7. **Ghrelin**—The growling hormone produced by the stomach that tells us we are hungry. If we skip or delay meals, then more ghrelin gets produced, and the result is that our appetite grows continually and we search for higher calorie dense foods. Hunger is stressful, and our food can be stressful too. Poor food choices, when we are hungry make us hungrier!

8. **Melatonin**—When the stress from food and environment continues to rise, raising cortisol, this can upset the sleep hormone melatonin, which has a natural cycle of when the body goes to sleep between the hours of 10:00 PM–6:00 AM. This is known as the circadian rhythm, and the melatonin-opposing hormone is cortisol. Sleeping well reduces stress, encourages human growth hormone to flow throughout the body between the hours of 10:00 PM and 2:00 AM, and encourages weight loss and fat burn. Sleeping between the hours of 2:00 AM and 6:00 AM encourages psychic repair and memory. We must strive to have 8 hours of un-interrupted sleep.

---

[8] Adamandia D. Kriketos, PhD, Seng Khee Gan, MBBS, FRACP, Ann M. Poynten, MBBS, FRACP, Stuart M. Furler, PHD, Donald J. Chisholm, MBBS, FRACP and Lesley V. Campbell, MBBS, FRACP, "Exercise Increases Adiponectin Levels and Insulin Sensitivity in Humans, *Diabetes Care* 27(2) (2004): 629–630.

STRESS LEVELS
Mental Stress
Pain Stress
Diet Stress

1 Cortisol/Adrenals starts weight gain

2 Insulin/Pancreas activates inflammation via sugar

3 Estrogen rises Testosterone weakens

4 Thyroid metabolism slows down

5 Leptin resistance more fat storage
FAT

HUNGER

6 Adiponectin fat feedback system shuts down

7 Ghrelin hunger signals increase

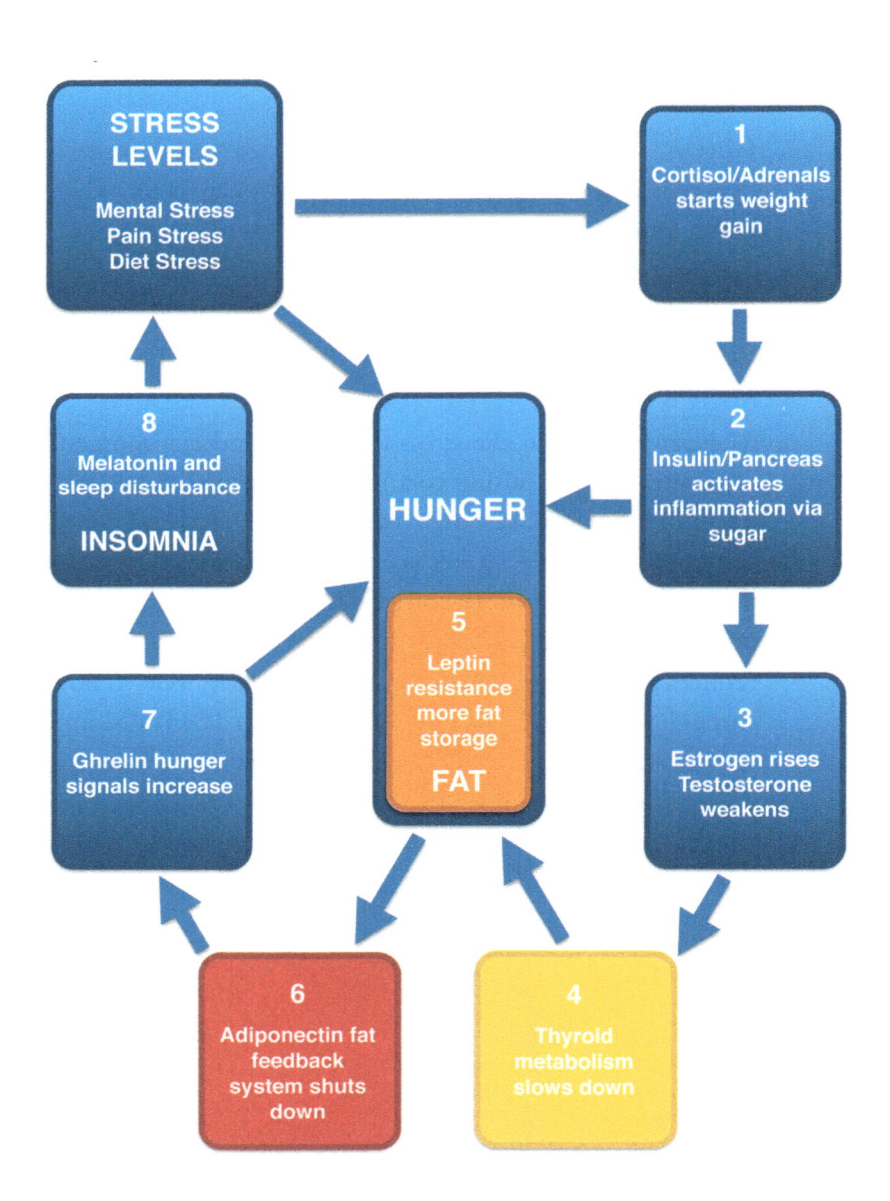

8 Melatonin and sleep disturbance
INSOMNIA

Stress, Hunger, and Weight Gain Cycle

❬ Stress, Hunger, and Weight Gain Cycle

1. **Cortisol**—High levels of this stress hormone release excess sugars into the blood, which are responsible for belly fat and weight gain.

2. **Insulin**—Excess blood sugar causes swings in the levels, and this irregularity causes inflammation, fat storage, and higher blood pressure.

3. **Estrogen**—Fat cells absorb sugar and increase in size, and they release estrogen. High levels cause fat storage on breasts, bellies, legs, and buttocks in both men and women.

4. **Thyroid**—High levels of estrogen and cortisol cause the thyroid gland to malfunction.

5. **Leptin**—Fat-cell signals become blocked by inflammation. Low levels of leptin or resistance cause the body to hold on to fat cells for longer.

6. **Adiponectin**—Fat-signaling system breaks down, and the fat cells become hungry for more sugar.

7. **Ghrelin**—Hunger signals increase and increase appetite for more food urgently.

8. **Melatonin**—Chronic stress and tension creates poor adrenal output, and as cortisol swings out of balance during the daytime, it throws off the nighttime sleep signal via melatonin levels becoming low.

Balance "the Fat Eight" Hormones for a Better Burn

The aforementioned hormones are all biochemically related to weight gain, obesity, and diabetes. Here's a quick overview on how to get these bad fat hormones under control by:

1. Your adrenal glands. Balance these with low-dose Pregnenolone/ DHEA therapy and glandular therapy. This will rev up your fat metabolism, balance cortisol / DHEA levels, and lower your high blood pressure. Altogether you'll get a deeper sleep, which helps to prevent Alzheimer's and relieve arthritis.

2. Your pancreas and its glucagon output (fat-burning hormone) and insulin (fat-storing hormone) levels. Balance these with low- to moderate-GI foods and enzymes.

3. Your sex hormones. Lower estrogen, balance progesterone, and elevate testosterone naturally to nurture the muscle-building process. This will automatically boost your fat burn, helping you to incinerate more calories. Progesterone therapy balances cortisol, calms the body, and improves sleep patterns and cognitive ability.

4. Your thyroid hormones. This gland and its hormones control the body's overall metabolic speed, rate of digestion, fat metabolism, and hair growth. Reverse T3 levels can be lowered using a thyroid drug called Cytomel (popular with the bodybuilding underground) combined with clenbuterol (adrenal steroid drug) however this is illegal for consumption in the USA? UK and Europe. This creates really lean bodybuilders with not an ounce of fat! The principles they use is to boost the thyroid and adrenal glands. Our natural and safer alternative is to supply the thyroid gland with iodine, kelp, selenium and balanced adrenal hormones and liver function.

5. Balancing leptin levels. Fat cells regulate *their size* with the hormone leptin. Leptin comes from the Greek word *leptos*,

which means "thin." Leptin is released from the fat cells when enough food has been consumed and the leptin shuts down the appetite center in the brain. A simple African fruit can really help rebuild the leptin levels and reset the appetite centre, with some healthy good food choices, that will get you to lose a lot of weight.

6. Adiponectin. This hormone helps to drive fat out of the cells of the body to help create sugar to be burnt as energy.

7. Ghrelin, the hunger hormone starts to behave itself due to regular meals and the effective use of good protein snacks in between meals.

8. Melatonin. Having balanced meals and balanced cortisol levels will allow the body to rest well at night to allow for repair and regeneration of the body's tissues. However, a really good night's sleep will encourage the body to burn fat[9].

The right way to create more energy is by rebooting your hormones and increasing the overall metabolism of the body. Choose your carbs carefully to encourage fat burning, melt the flab off, and iron out your insulin, cortisol, and estrogen issues. Bad carbs can cause leptin resistance and an increase in appetite. Sugars make you hungry for more sugar.

Some diets allow the use of whole grains, corn, and yeast-based foods. In this book we take the no-nonsense, no-grain approach. Omitting heavy foods such as corn, rice, wheat, bread, and pastry is important because these are high–glycemic index foods and can contain yeast, which is now understood to cause weight gain[10]

---

[9] Maria Alonso-Vale, Isabel Cardoso, et al, "Melatonin and the circadian entrainment of metabolic and hormonal activities in primary isolated adipocytes," *Journal of Pineal Research* 45.4 (2008): 422–429.

[10] H. Weker, "Simple obesity in children. A study on the role of nutritional factors," Medycyna Wieku Rozwojowego – *Developmental Period Medicine*. 10(1) (2006): 3–191. http://www.ncbi.nlm.nih.gov/pubmed/16733288

and diabetes[11]. High–glycemic index grains made together with yeast can cause a lot of metabolic problems.

Putting It All Together

1. With the support of reducing dietary stress, eating balanced meals, and eating small amounts of food regularly (every three hours), the pancreas balances out the blood sugars, which in turn balances out cortisol and raises DHEA and Pregnenolone.

2. Improved DHEA and Pregnenolone levels boost the sex hormones testosterone and progesterone, which in turn switches on the thyroid gland.

3. The thyroid gland, feeling the effects of all the adrenal and sex-hormone glands working properly, will now push the body into fat-burn mode by helping to boost the metabolism through the conversion of thyroid hormone T4 into the more potent T3.

4. As the fat burns, leptin sensitivity returns and effortless weight loss continues as long as the pancreatic insulin function stays stable, hence the need to test blood sugars, HbA1c, C-reactive protein, and triglycerides regularly to make sure these are optimal. The African mango *Irvingia gabonensis* and *Gymnema Sylvestre* are instrumental in building this bridge naturally.

5. Leptin sensitivity is now restored, the feedback between the amount of fat being stored and the brain monitoring the amount that's stored is now functioning, and the individual starts to burn excessive stored fat reserves. As the leptin loop

---

11   M. O'Connor, D. Kiely, M. Mulvihil, A. Winters, et al, "School Nutrition Survey," *Ir Medical Journal* 86(3) (1993); 89–91. http://www.ncbi.nlm.nih.gov/pubmed/8567245

stimulates cells to release fats, the adiponectin gets released too, increasing metabolism.

6. Adiponectin reboots the pancreas and restores insulin sensitivity by choosing the correct carbs, proteins, green veggies, and regular meals.

7. Adiponectin encourages your muscle's ability to use carbohydrates for energy, stimulates your metabolism, and increases the rate at which your body breaks down fat; and to add to that, it curbs your appetite by reducing ghrelin levels.

8. Ghrelin levels reduce when the person has balanced sugar control and regular meals with good sources of protein.

9. As the sugar levels balance and the protein is regularly consumed, the ghrelin hunger signal switches off, and this in turn allows melatonin to allow the body to sleep well.

Leptin/adiponectin are the key. These are the hormones that can make or break your diet goals. The leptin/adiponectin hormone helps you understand that appetite can be controlled by allowing your brain to recognize that you are full and that you have good fat-cell feedback.

By regulating your dietary sugars and carbohydrates carefully, taking daily Irvingia and Gymnema, improving your leptin sensitivity, and raising your adiponectin levels, you can shed weight/body fat fast, by fixing the human appetite signal system.

Any diet program that does not consider these two key fat-burning hormones will cause your body's fat metabolism eventually to stall, and then frustration sets in, which is another emotional stressor that affects our adrenals again.

THE TESTING

Chapter 4

Testing Your Eight Fat-Causing Hormones

Our hormones dictate our body shape. Our hormones control the ratio between muscle and fat, and specifically our hormones deposit fat in very specific areas—cortisol creates belly fat, insulin issues create the muffin top, and estrogens create bigger breasts and butts in both men and women. Male boobs (gynecomastia) appear and female breasts become enlarged because estrogen makes them grow. Estrogen as a hormone will stimulate fat deposition and breast growth in any mammal.

If you feed estrogen to cows (plus take them off grass and give them corn and BGH/antibiotics), they will gain weight, and that's precisely what farmers do to make a better sale price for the animal. The opposite of estrogen is testosterone; it burns fat and builds muscle.

Estrogen stresses and creates leptin resistance, and this blocks any form of significant fat burn. The system is then *stuck* on weight gain because the appetite signals have been activated into signaling hunger and the search for food and calories.

Excess sugar in the blood will be managed by insulin, and this hormone will deposit fat on the muffin-top area, and unbalanced cortisol levels create the cortisol belly (from emotional stress, dietary allergies, and physical pain and inflammation).
You should start finding out some really good information about the fat eight as follows:

1. **Cortisol**
   - Adrenal blood chemistry scores
   - Take the stress questionnaire
   - Do you have a parasite living in your body (bugs or yeast)?

- Do you have any allergies?
- Adrenal cortex stress profile interpretation

2. **Insulin**
- Fasting blood sugar and HbA1c test

3. **Estrogen**
- Take the estrogen-dominance questionnaire
- Take the progesterone questionnaire
- Take the testosterone questionnaire
- Blood tests/hormone panels

4. **Thyroid**
- Body-temperature test and chart (see appendix)
- Iodine-patch test
- Take the thyroid questionnaire
- Optimal thyroid blood ranges

5. **Leptin**
- Take the blood sugar 3 hours after meals
- Take an HbA1c test
- Measure your CRP
- Check your cholesterol and triglycerides
- Men—measure your testosterone for levels too low
- Women—measure for high DHEA and low progesterone
- Measure your thyroid-stimulating hormone (TSH)

6. **Adiponectin**
- Adiponectin testing is performed on a blood sample drawn from a vein by your MD or DO or at your local private blood chemistry lab.
- Additional tests may include glucose, insulin levels, Glucose Tolerance Test, Hemoglobin A1c, C-peptide, leptin, lipid profile, liver profile, and CRP.

7. **Ghrelin**
- This can be tested by your MD or DO or at your local private blood-chemistry lab.

8. Melatonin
- A simple saliva test done at home can measure levels of melatonin within the body. The test is usually performed in the evening just before the usual bedtime, around 9:30–10:30 PM. It can be combined with the adrenal hormone test at the same time, as the saliva will reflect nocturnal melatonin levels.

CHAPTER 5

Testing Cortisol Levels

How do your adrenals cope with stress?

This information will allow you to start taking the right amount of Pregnenolone to support your recovering adrenals. There are several tests that can be done. Some are simple and slightly inaccurate and variable, and others are much more accurate, such as the Functional Adrenal Stress Profile (201 or 205V) from BioHealth labs in the USA.

1. Simple Adrenal Testing

You'll need some physiology data from your local physician to do this part, or you can even do it at home if you know how to use a blood-pressure monitor. These are just clues and not diagnostic.

Basic Adrenal guidelines[1]:

- Low blood pressure = Low Blood pressure = less than 100/60 = low adrenal gland function/hypoadrenia/Pregnenolone/DHEA deficient/low electrolytes
- Normal blood pressure = stable adrenals
- High blood pressure = overstimulated adrenals/acute stress/hyperadrenia/usually Pregnenolone/DHEA deficient/excess electrolytes (excess salt)

---
1   Steve Denk, "Physicians Training Material Flow Systems Analysis" *Biomedx.com,* ," Chicago, Illinois July 2003.

Treatment = monitor trending

- Low blood pressure—increase electrolytes, salt, potassium, calcium, and licorice
- Normal blood pressure—no treatment, take regular potassium-based foods for health maintenace
- High blood pressure—electrolyte excess, reduce salt and calcium, and increase magnesium and potassium/ginseng (*no* licorice).

N.B The above interpretation is only a guide; please check with your physician.

2. Blood Chemistry Adrenal Testing

You can also gauge how the adrenal glands are doing by looking at your sodium and potassium levels. These levels are regulated by the adrenal glands, which can rev up hormone production. You simply cannot get into a fat burn mode if the adrenals are dysfunctional.

Potassium Levels[2]

Potassium levels need to be checked if you experience the following:
- Muscle weakness
- Fatigue
- Mental confusion
- Heart disturbances
- Problems in nerve conduction

BLOOD POTASSIUM	STANDARD US UNITS	STANDARD INTERNATIONAL UNITS
CONVENTIONAL LABORATORY RANGE	3.5 - 5.3 mEq/L	3.5 - 5.3 mmol/L
OPTIMAL RANGE	4.0 - 4.5 mEq/L	4.0 - 4.5 mmol/L
ALARM RANGE	< 3.0 or > 6.0 mEq/L	< 3.0 or > 6.0 mmol/L

2   Dicken Weatherby, ND, and Scott Ferguson, ND, Blood Chemistry and CBC Analysis-Clinical lab testing from a functional perspective, (Vis Medicatrix Press, Oregon : *Bear Mountain Publishing*, 2002)

Potassium level Interpretation:

If the adrenals are *hypoactive*, potassium will be high.

Hypo-Adrenal Signs:

- Low blood pressure
- Craving for salt
- Chronic fatigue
- Afternoon yawning
- Weakness and dizziness
- Extreme fatigue after exercise
- Poor circulation
- Weakness after colds and flu

If the adrenals are *hyperactive*, potassium will be low.

Hyper-Adrenal signs:

- High blood pressure
- Headaches
- Hot flashes
- Excessive hair growth on face or body (females)
- Keyed up, trouble calming down
- Clenching and grinding teeth

Sodium Levels[3]

Although nothing replaces a good lab test result and the advice and guidance of a competent physician, there are clues to the conditions of an adrenal disorder. Sodium levels have to fall within a certain optimal zone and are chiefly controlled by the adrenal cortex hormones, especially by a hormone called aldosterone.

---

3   Dicken Weatherby, ND, and Scott Ferguson, ND, Blood Chemistry and CBCAnalysis-Clinical lab testing from a Functional Perspective, (Vis Medicatrix Press, Oregon : *Bear Mountain Publishing*, 2002)

Blood Sodium	Standard US Units	Standard International Units
Conventional Laboratory Range	135 - 145 mEq/L	135 - 145 mmol/L
Optimal Range	135 - 142 mEq/L	135 - 142 mmol/L
Alarm Range	< 125 or > 155 mEq/L	< 125 or > 155 mmol/L

Sodium Level Interpretation:

If the sodium is high, it indicates adrenal hyperfunction.
- High blood pressure
- Headaches
- Hot flashes
- Excessive hair growth on face or body (females)
- Keyed up, trouble calming down
- Clenching and grinding teeth

If the sodium is low, it indicates adrenal hypo-function.
- Low blood pressure
- Craving for salt
- Chronic fatigue
- Afternoon yawning
- Weakness and dizziness
- Extreme fatigue after exercise
- Poor circulation
- Weakness after colds and flu

Review the signs of adrenal hyperfunction and hypo-function on the preceding pages.

N.B The above interpretation is only an educational guide; please check with your regular competent physician to validate.

3. Social Stress Questionnaire[4]

Emotional pulls and strains can cause our adrenals to become weaker. We feel stressed when we eat too many carbs, just like

LIFE EVENT	YES	NO	POINT VALUE	SCORE
DEATH OF A SPOUSE			100	
DIVORCE			75	
MARITAL SEPARATION			65	
JAIL TERM			63	
DEATH OF A CLOSE FAMILY MEMBER			63	
DISMISSED FROM WORK			53	
RETIREMENT			47	
CHANGE IN FAMILY MEMBERS HEALTH			44	
RESPONSIBLE FOR CAREGIVING			44	
PREGNANCY			40	
SEXUAL DIFFICULTIES			39	
CHANGE IN FINANCIAL STATUS			38	
DEATH OF A CLOSE FRIEND			37	
BUSINESS READJUSTMENT			36	
MORTGAGE IN EXCESS OF $250,000			31	
FORECLOSURE			30	
CHANGE IN WORK RESPONSIBILITY			29	
OFFSPRING LEAVING HOME			29	
DISCORD WITH IN-LAWS			29	
OUTSTANDING PERSONAL ACHIEVEMENT			28	
SPOUSE COMMENCES OR CEASES EMPLOYMENT			26	
COMMENCING OR FINISHING SCHOOL			26	
CHANGE IN LIVING CONDITIONS			25	
DISCORD WITH EMPLOYER			23	
CHANGE IN WORK HOURS			20	
TOTAL SCORE				

---

4   T. H. Holmes and R. H. Rahe, "Adaptation of The Social Readjustment rating scale," *Journal of Psychosomatic Research* 11(2) (1967), 213–221.

we feel stressed when we watch a horror movie, but we must work to reduce this "social stress." Figure out your worst social stressors:

Interpretation:

Score < 150 = 37% chance of illness in the next year
Score >150–299 = 50% chance of illness
Score >300 = 80% chance of illness
How did you score?

Are your social stresses getting too much?
Can you reduce the level?
Have you considered meditation and yoga?
What can you do or control that will help you to relax and unwind?

4. Adrenocortex Stress Profile

This is the *best test* to really comprehend what the adrenals are doing, especially as it tells you how the levels of cortisol and stress change through a twenty-four-hour cycle.

Figuring out how well your adrenals are working through the day with an Adrenocortex Stress Profile is so powerful. This is a saliva test kit that can be ordered from BioHealth lab, listed in the appendix. They will send you the test kit so you can take the samples at home or at work, freeze them, fill out your paperwork, and return the test-kit samples to the lab. They should be able to run the test within seven to ten days, and you and your physician can discuss the results or you can book a Skype appointment with my clinic.

Let's explain the meaning of this chart. There are three stages of the adrenal response, and they are listed as follows:

Stage 1—*Alarm response:* As the stressor is identified, the body produces adrenaline to affect the fight, fright, or flight

Progression of Stages of Adrenal Exhaustion

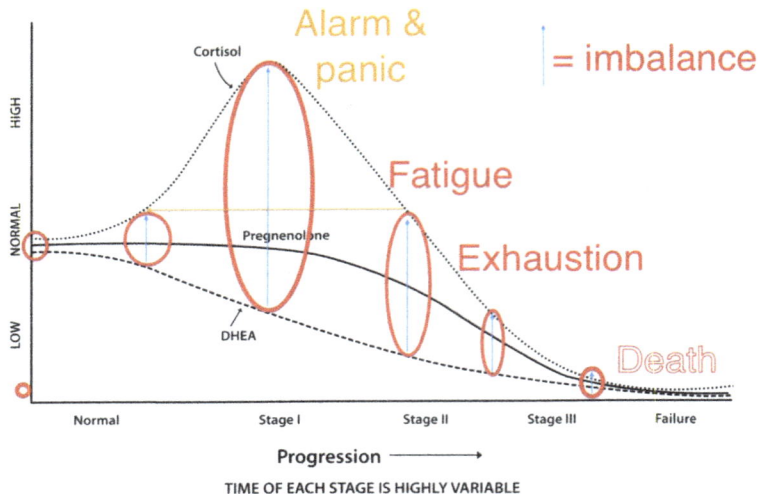

Graph showing Cortisol, Pregnenolone, and DHEA hormone levels across Normal, Stage I (Alarm & panic), Stage II (Fatigue), Stage III (Exhaustion), and Failure (Death) stages. = imbalance

TIME OF EACH STAGE IS HIGHLY VARIABLE

Stages of adrenal exhaustion over time showing three hormone levels.

response. Cortisol is also produced. Intense negative emotions, parasite infections, poor diet, pain, and trauma will cause the cortisol to rise/spike and create the beginnings of weight gain if the stressors are not reduced.

Stage 2—*Fatigue or Resistance response:* As the stressor continues and the body starts to tire from the persistent output of adrenal hormones, the levels of hormones start to decline, due to the adrenal gland tissues becoming weaker and the negative effects on the human body become noticeable.

Stage 3—*Burnout and Exhaustion:* The body's resources are depleted to a point where physically you are totally exhausted and the adrenal hormone production dwindles to very low levels and the immune system starts to fail and pathologies are apparent.

Stage 4—*Failure of the adrenals:* This will cause a system or organ failure probably resulting in death. This stage is associated with severe advanced adrenal crisis (Addisonian crisis? Cushing's crisis?) or acute adrenal depletion, which in turn can cause symptoms of sudden, penetrating pain in the lower back or kidney pain, severe vomiting, diarrhea, dehydration and electrolyte loss, low blood pressure, and loss of consciousness.

Some of the symptoms of stress are eczema, headaches, weight gain, irritability, anger issues, diabetes, osteoporosis, cardiovascular symptoms, autoimmune disease, chronic fatigue, Alzheimer's, and cancer.

Cortisol dysfunction can cause several problems, which are usually addressed by MDs only through the symptomatic medication, when really the adrenals need to be tested and supported, where needed, with the appropriate natural hormones.

It is the relative distance *between* the cortisol and the DHEA that creates weight gain and fatigue and slows your thyroid and metabolism. This is indicated by the cortisol-DHEA ratio.

The following patient test results show that he/she is in Stage 3 burnout.

BioHealth

Kit 201 BioHealth labs, California, USA

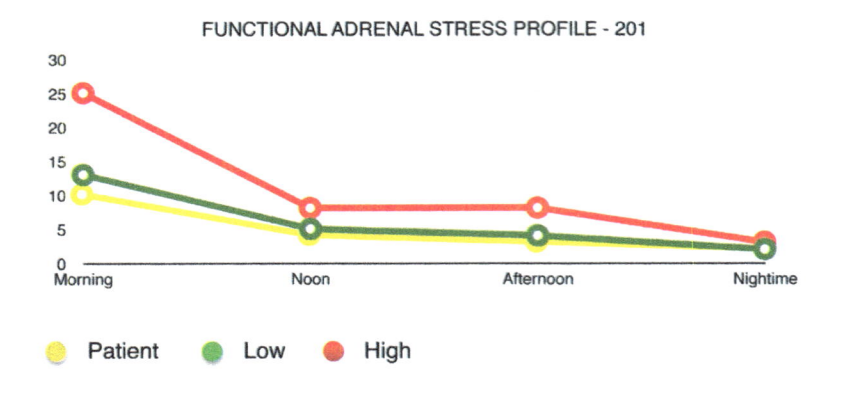

FUNCTIONAL ADRENAL STRESS PROFILE - 201

● Patient ● Low ● High

	Result	Reference Range	Units
Cortisol - Morning (6-8AM)	10.1*	13.0-24.0	nM/L
Cortisol - Noon (12-1PM)	3.1*	5.0-8.0	nM/L
Cortisol - Afternoon (4-5PM)	2.7*	4.0-7.0	nM/L
Cortisol - Night Time (10PM-12AM)	1.4	1.0-3.0	nM/L
Cortisol Sum	17.3*	23.0-42.0	nM/L
DHEA-S Average	2.84	2.00-10.00	ng/mL
Cortisol/DHEA-S Ratio	6.1	5.0-6.0	Ratio

Test sample—the Functional Adrenal Stress Profile (Stage 3 burnout).

- The ideal cortisol sum is between 36 and 42. Ideal DHEA is 6 or higher.
- If your cortisol sum is greater than 42 and the DHEA is less than 6, then you are in Stage 1- hyperadrenia and the alarm response.
- If your cortisol sum is normal and the DHEA is lower than 6, then you are in Stage 2—the fatigue response.
- If your cortisol sum and DHEA are both low, then you are in Stage 3 – exhaustion or burn-out.

It is the relative distance between the cortisol and the DHEA that creates weight gain and fatigue and slows your thyroid and metabolism. This is indicated by the cortisol-DHEA ratio. The preceding patient test results show that he/she is in Stage 3 burnout.

N.B Treatment—Some natural hormones might have to be prescribed in order to achieve optimal results, however you need the guidance of a competent physician trained in bioidentical hormone therapy.

Cortisol Stress, Parasites, Allergies, and Weight Gain

Diseases associated with cortisol dysfunction are as follows: ear, nose, and throat allergies[5]; food allergies; asthma[6]; infections; obesity[7]; schizophrenia; osteoporosis; anxiety; depression; chronic fatigue; diabetes; anorexia; cardiovascular diseases; and cancer.

Parasites, bacteria, yeast, and allergies will raise cortisol levels. Parasites, bacteria, yeast, and allergies are stressful, right? Fat people unknowingly have chronic bacterial infections, which can induce their obesity[8]. One in particular has been clearly linked with weight gain, and it's called Enterobacter cloacae B29[9]. Killing the bacterial overgrowth induces serious weight

---

5   L. Chatzi, M. Torrent, I. Romieu, et al. "Diet, wheeze, and atopy in school children in Menorca, Spain," *Pediatric Allergy Immunology* 18(6) (2007): 480–485.

6   Fitzpatrick, S., R. Joks, and J. I. Silverberg. "Obesity is associated with increased asthma severity and exacerbations, and increased serum immunoglobulin E in inner-city adults." *Clinical & Experimental Allergy* 42, no. 5 (2012): 747-759.

7   Ibid 57

8   Matej Bajzer and Randy J. Seeley, "Physiology: Obesity and gut flora," *Nature* 444 (2006): 1009–1010.

9   "An opportunistic pathogen isolated from the gut of an obese human causes obesity in germfree mice," *The ISME Journal* (2012).[Missing info-author name(s), volume, page numbers]

loss. Parasites, too, can cause weight gain and obesity according to some scientists[10].

People also can consume foods they're allergic to, sometimes on a daily basis. When this happens, your body responds with stress[11], which triggers the release of cortisol[12]. And this in turn screws up the blood's sugar levels and makes us put on weight.

> **KEY POINT: Cortisol is a *glucocorticosteroid*, and when it is secreted during any stress (psychological, physical, or physiological), the blood sugar will be forced to rise.**

This cortisol release upsets the regulation of sugars because "stress" causes the body to release more sugar to the muscles when they enter the flight, fright, or fight mode.

As blood-sugar levels repeatedly rise, like a roller coaster the pancreas will also grow tired over time, and its ability to handle sugars goes into decline. This sets the stage for diabetes and weight gain. Allergies (also known as antigens) create antibodies within the blood. Antibodies are the body's response to allergies so it can recognize the difference between self and nonself.

While your body is creating antibodies against parasites, food allergies, and toxins, you're also making reactive chemical substances such as histamines, cytokines, lymphokines, and interferon. These substances act like hormones and as such create dramatic effects on physiology, which can have profound effects on the human nervous system, glandular systems of the thyroid and adrenals, and immune system.

Parasites, food, and environmental toxins have been connected to a wide range of medical conditions from mild symptoms of gastric reflux to very serious diseases such as heart diseases and

---

10   http://undergroundhealthreporter.com/causes-of-obesity#axzz2rYgnaeB0

11   F. Stenius, M. Borres, M. Bottai, et al, "Salivary cortisol levels and allergy in children: the ALADDIN birth cohort," *Journal of Allergy Clinical Immunology* 128(6) (2011): 1335–1339.

12   A. Buske-Kirschbaum, "Cortisol responses to stress in allergic children: interaction with the immune response," *Neuro-immunomodulation* 16(5) (2009): 325–332.

cancer. Allergies have also been openly associated with migraines, depression, arthritis, and chronic fatigue immunodeficiency syndrome.

Common Parasite Symptoms

- Chronic allergies
- Dark circles under eyes
- Gas
- Bloating
- Belching
- Chronic constipation or diarrhea
- Burning anus
- Itchy anus
- Difficulty losing weight
- Difficulty gaining weight
- Chronic fatigue
- Depression
- ADD
- ADHD
- Colitis (Crohn's/ulcerative)

Testing for Parasites

There are two key tests that basically prove if you have a parasite infection.

One method assesses your immune system, and the other actually gathers specimens taken from the stool itself.

1. **Complete Blood Count (CBC)**—Check the monocyte percentages. They should be less than 7 percent. The average MD is trained to use a range of greater than 13 percent, but healthy, uninfected, trouble-free guts are below 7 percent. Test the eosinophils, as they ideally should be less

than 3 percent. This test will *not* tell you the name of the parasite, it only tells you if you have one or not. If it's any higher than 7 percent or 3 percent, go and do a comprehensive stool-analysis test.

2. **Comprehensive Digestive Stool Analysis**—This test uses fresh stool samples, over three or four bowel movements, sent to a lab for thorough examination. Once you have the name of the parasite, inform your physician and ask more advice about better ways to eradicate a parasite. Botanical treatments such as very low doses of clove, artemesia, black walnut, and oregano oil are excellent at removing parasites. Treatment time is usually sixty to ninety days. Repeat CBC and stool test to confirm that the parasite has gone. Heavy parasite infection might need the intervention of a pharmaceutical drug (see MD or DO).

Risk Factors for Picking Up Parasites

- Eating food with unwashed hands
- Nail-biting
- Picking nose
- Eating food in unsanitary conditions
- Swallowing lake, river water
- Foreign travel
- Owning pets
- Drinking untreated water
- Eating raw fish or meat

Treatment for Parasites

Most parasite infections can be treated with botanicals and medications very successfully. Heavy infections require stronger medication (Flagyl, antibiotics); however, there are side effects associated with this action, such as liver-detox strains and candida infections.

Good botanicals such as wormwood, black walnut extract, cloves, pumpkin seeds, oregano oil, and diatomaceous earth are excellent at removing bad bugs from the body (bacteria, yeast, and parasites). Usually an antiparasite program lasts for sixty to ninety days and requires retesting the stool and CBC to really witness the absence of the parasites and that they have been clearly expelled from the digestive tract.

Treatment for Pathogenic Bacterial Parasites

Most bacterial infections can be treated using botanicals very successfully. Silver colloid is a good bacteriostatic and can be used in shorter intervals. Oregano oil is excellent. Condurango Blend is another top choice for scrubbing the bugs out. However, once the bugs have been eradicated over sixty days, then it is important to replace the missing friendly bacteria.

Treatment for Candida Yeast Parasite

Follow a no-sugar, no-grain diet while at the same time using an anti-yeast supplement. This will starve and kill the yeast overgrowth. Taking regular daily antifungal supplements is essential to scrubbing out the yeast. Further details are in my first book, *The Hidden Cure*.

Testing for Allergies

There are many advanced diagnostic labs that can perform detailed allergy screening. The method that we employ here at our clinic is based on discovering both immediate allergies using an IgE marker and delayed allergy marker using IgG. This way we erase all doubt about which foods create allergies and stress and which foods allow you to heal.

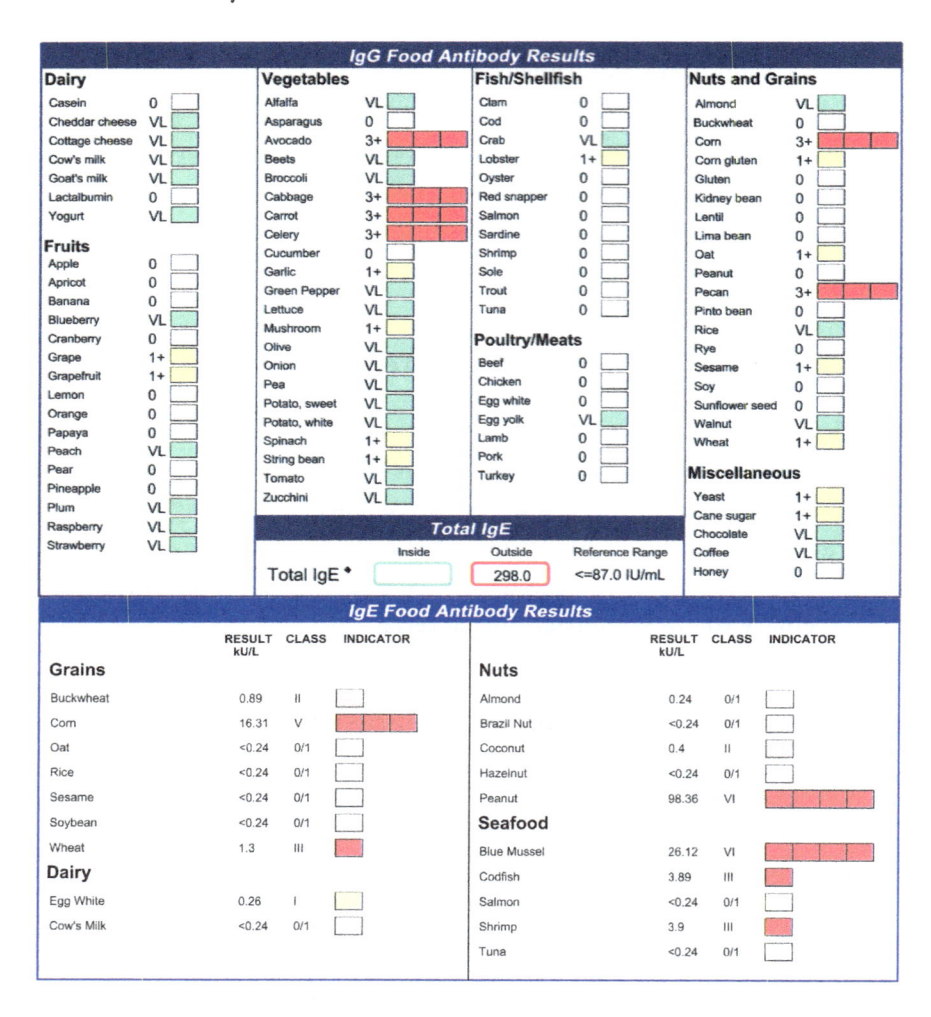

IgG Food Antibody Results

Dairy			Vegetables			Fish/Shellfish			Nuts and Grains		
Casein	0		Alfalfa	VL		Clam	0		Almond	VL	
Cheddar cheese	VL		Asparagus	0		Cod	0		Buckwheat	0	
Cottage cheese	VL		Avocado	3+		Crab	VL		Corn	3+	
Cow's milk	VL		Beets	VL		Lobster	1+		Corn gluten	1+	
Goat's milk	VL		Broccoli	VL		Oyster	0		Gluten	0	
Lactalbumin	0		Cabbage	3+		Red snapper	0		Kidney bean	0	
Yogurt	VL		Carrot	3+		Salmon	0		Lentil	0	
Fruits			Celery	3+		Sardine	0		Lima bean	0	
Apple	0		Cucumber	0		Shrimp	0		Oat	1+	
Apricot	0		Garlic	1+		Sole	0		Peanut	0	
Banana	0		Green Pepper	VL		Trout	0		Pecan	3+	
Blueberry	VL		Lettuce	VL		Tuna	0		Pinto bean	0	
Cranberry	0		Mushroom	1+					Rice	VL	
Grape	1+		Olive	VL		**Poultry/Meats**			Rye	0	
Grapefruit	1+		Onion	VL		Beef	0		Sesame	1+	
Lemon	0		Pea	VL		Chicken	0		Soy	0	
Orange	0		Potato, sweet	VL		Egg white	0		Sunflower seed	0	
Papaya	0		Potato, white	VL		Egg yolk	VL		Walnut	VL	
Peach	VL		Spinach	1+		Lamb	0		Wheat	1+	
Pear	0		String bean	1+		Pork	0		**Miscellaneous**		
Pineapple	0		Tomato	VL		Turkey	0		Yeast	1+	
Plum	VL		Zucchini	VL					Cane sugar	1+	
Raspberry	VL								Chocolate	VL	
Strawberry	VL								Coffee	VL	
									Honey	0	

Total IgE: Inside — , Outside — 298.0, Reference Range <=87.0 IU/mL

IgE Food Antibody Results

	RESULT kU/L	CLASS	INDICATOR
Grains			
Buckwheat	0.89	II	
Corn	16.31	V	
Oat	<0.24	0/1	
Rice	<0.24	0/1	
Sesame	<0.24	0/1	
Soybean	<0.24	0/1	
Wheat	1.3	III	
Dairy			
Egg White	0.26	I	
Cow's Milk	<0.24	0/1	

	RESULT kU/L	CLASS	INDICATOR
Nuts			
Almond	0.24	0/1	
Brazil Nut	<0.24	0/1	
Coconut	0.4	II	
Hazelnut	<0.24	0/1	
Peanut	98.36	VI	
Seafood			
Blue Mussel	26.12	VI	
Codfish	3.89	III	
Salmon	<0.24	0/1	
Shrimp	3.9	III	
Tuna	<0.24	0/1	

Sample report of an IgE and IgG allergy test from Genova Diagnostics labs.

IgE-mediated responses are histamine-related, and as such, when MDs encounter a suspected allergy in a patient, they usually prescribe an antihistamine.

There is a large amount of medical research that supports such a strategy. However, my opinion is to find out what the offending allergy is by screening the IgE antibodies carefully to understand the immediate allergy and subsequently to avoid it. Asthma, hives, and eczema are mostly IgE-mediated allergy responses. Patients must find out what substances they are allergic to rather than just treating the symptoms.

IgG-mediated responses are delayed responses and involve a reaction within the cells. The antigen binds to the cell, and this activates an immune response against the cell. For example, if you have B or AB blood (which means you're allergic to chicken) and you eat chicken on Sunday, you won't get the allergy response (acid reflux or a migraine) until days later. Most MDs do not check for IgG responses; however, medical literature supports the fact that 80 percent of allergy responses are IgG or delayed responses.

If you don't find out what the delayed allergies are, then once the adrenals become stressed (cortisol) repeatedly, this has the domino effect of hurting the pancreas (insulin resistance) and setting you up for weight gain and immune problems that could, over decades, lead to heart disease or even worse—cancer. Stress can adversely cause your glucose and insulin ratio to be profoundly upset with the ultimate effect of slowing down the metabolism. Cortisol stimulates the deposit of fat, the accelerated breakdown of muscles and joints, and induces sleeping problems such as insomnia.

The question is: what are the allergies that make you fat? Is it food? Chocolate, coffee, dairy, eggs, or wheat? Is it dust mites? Mold?

Ask your holistic-minded physician to order a full 120 foods and inhalants panel for IgE and IgG. Follow the process and avoid eating those foods and dwelling in those environments.

Your physician will need to take a blood sample from you in order to process the test. Understanding what substances you are allergic to will make tremendous health improvements and step up your metabolism for the better. When your metabolism is working better, you will look better and live longer!

Gluten-Allergy and Wheat-Sensitivity Questionnaire

Bread and cereals cause obesity[13] in children[14] and atherosclerosis[15] in adults. Bread is one of those yeasty food items that we eat all the time, during any season—for breakfast, lunch, snacks, and dinner. Modern sliced bread contains very few nutrients due to the processing of the flour, which is why most bread has to be enriched with vitamins[16]. Enriched flour products tend to be higher on the glycemic index, quickly raising blood-sugar levels.

Bread, having a high glycemic index (meaning it has a high sugar content), taxes the pancreas enormously, as it has to produce a rapid insulin response. A rapid insulin response is the body's way of controlling the sudden shift in blood-sugar levels as a result of the bread's consumption.

If someone habitually eats junk food (wheat, sugar, flour, processed meat, artificial milkshakes, etc.), he or she causes swings in insulin, and as a result the pancreas gets "tired." If the junk food has yeast in it, or if that person is taking a course of antibiotics, then trouble will brew, literally.

---

13 M. O'Connor, D. Kiely, M. Mulvihil, A. Winters, et al, "School Nutrition Survey," Irish Medical Journal 86(3) (1993): 89–91. http://www.ncbi.nlm.nih.gov/pubmed/8567245

14 H. Weker, "Simple obesity in children. A study on the role of nutritional factors," Medycyna Wieku Rozwojowego 10(1) (2006): 3–191. http://www.ncbi.nlm.nih.gov/pubmed/16733288

15 Cecil M. Burchfiel, Dwayne M. Reed, Ellen B. Marcus, Jack P. Strong, and Takuji Hayashi, "Association of Diabetes Mellitus with Coronary Atherosclerosis and Myocardial Lesions: An Autopsy Study from the Honolulu Heart Program," *American Journal of Epidemiology* 137(12) (1993): 1328–1340.

16 Enriched Flour - http://en.wikipedia.org/wiki/Enriched_flour; accessed April 2012.

If you follow a gluten-free diet, you will be able to stabilize your blood sugar, gain improved liver function and energy levels, have less migraines and neuropathies, have less eczema, reduce and remove cravings, have better bowel movements, get more sleep, and also become slimmer. Some early research shows that a yeast-free/gluten-free/casein-free diet has wonderful benefits for autism and other neurological diseases[17].

Gluten sensitivity and celiac disease are a known cause of scleroderma, rheumatoid[18], lupus, and other autoimmune diseases. Even if other tests for gluten sensitivity and celiac disease are negative or inconclusive, trial of a gluten-free and casein-free (GFCF) diet should be considered[19]. If you score moderate to high numbers on the following questionnaire, you should be yeast-, gluten-, and wheat-free for two to three months. This will allow your guts to heal from the allergic response to yeast/wheat within the gut lining.

Are You Sensitive to Wheat and Gluten?

Scroll down the list and see if you suffer from any of the following symptoms (refer to chart on next page).

Now count up how many "yes" answers you have and check your total against the table below:

0 to 4   It is likely you are not gluten or wheat sensitive.

5 to 10 There is the possibility of a small issue, increasing with each "yes."

---

17   J. H. Elder, "The gluten-free, casein-free diet in autism: an overview with clinical implications," Nutr Clin Pract 23(6) (2008): 583–588.[Missing info-full journal name]

18   M. Hvatum, L. Kanerud, R. Hällgren, and P. Brandtzaeg, "The gut–joint axis: cross reactive food antibodies in rheumatoid arthritis," Gut 55(9) (2006): 1240–1247.

19   Charlene Laino, "Celiac Disease Underdiagnosed?" WebMD Health News, May 20, 2008 - http://www.webmd.com/digestive-disorders/celiac-disease/news/20080520/celiac-disease- underdiagnosed

> 11 There is a definite problem, and it's recommended to cut out all wheat and gluten foods for at least three months. Follow a low-GI diet immediately.

ARE YOU SENSITIVE TO WHEAT AND GLUTEN?	YES	NO
DIFFICULTY GAINING WEIGHT/ANOREXIC		
DIFFICULTY LOSING WEIGHT		
WEIGHT GAIN		
TENDENCY TO BECOME INTOXICATED EASILY		
GASSY AFTER EATING DAIRY PRODUCTS		
HAVE OTHER FOOD ALLERGIES		
SUFFER FROM HEADACHES/MIGRAINES		
SUFFER FROM JOINT PAIN/SWOLLEN JOINTS		
SUFFER FROM HORMONE IMBALANCES/MOOD SWINGS		
BURPY/WINDY/GASSY		
RASHES ON SKIN		
BLOATED STOMACH AFTER CERTAIN FOODS		
CRAMPING PAINS IN THE ABDOMEN		
CRAVE SWEETS & CANDY		
OVEREATS CARBOHYDRATES & SWEETS		
OVERLY SENSITIVE/CRIES EASILY		
CHRONIC FATIGUE		
DIABETES/SUGAR ISSUES		
ANAEMIA		
CANDIDA/YEAST INFECTIONS		
DEPRESSION/LOW MOOD		
TOTAL SCORE		

Treatment for Allergies

This basically involves avoiding the known allergies (IgE and IgG) for a period of sixty to ninety days to allow the immune system to desensitize. Follow a rotation diet and steer clear of any allergic foods, beverages, and spices that one might be allergic to.

Yeast Infection Questionnaire:

Do you have a current yeast infection? If you think not, check anyway. Take the questionnaire (see chart on following page). Are you sensitive to yeast and candida? Scroll down the list and see if you suffer from any of the following symptoms.

Now count up how many "yes" answers you have and check your total against the following table:

0 to 3   It's likely you are not yeast sensitive.

3 to 5   It's possible there is a small issue, increasing with each "yes."

> 5   You definitely have a problem, and it's recommended to cut out all yeast foods for at least three months.

THE TOTAL FAT CURE

ARE YOU SENSITIVE TO YEAST & CANDIDA?	YES	NO
SKIN RASHES, ECZEMA/CRUSTINESS BEHIND EARS		
ITCHY SKIN/HIVES		
VAGINAL DISCHARGE		
ITCHY, BURNING PAINFUL SEX		
MASSIVE SUGAR CRAVINGS		
CRAVINGS FOR ALCOHOL		
BAD BREATH (HALITOSIS)		
WHITE COATED TONGUE		
RECURRING MOUTH ULCERS		
NAIL BED FUNGUS		
LIVER SPOTS, SKIN FUNGUS		
HEADACHE, HANGOVER		
GAS & BLOATING		
PAINFUL URINATION		
WHITE FLAKY MATTER IN THE EAR CANAL		
ACNE		
ASTHMA, SHORTNESS OF BREATH		
GASTRIC REFLUX/GERD/GASTRITIS		
CANCER (BREAST/UTERINE/PROSTATE)		
FIBROCYSTIC BREAST DISEASE		
DIABETES TYPE 2		
HIGH CHOLESTEROL		
GALLSTONES		
SINUSITIS		
AUTOIMMUNE DISEASES		
DEPRESSION/PANIC ATTACKS		
MENTAL CONFUSION		
HYPOTHYROIDISM AND, OF COURSE, WEIGHT GAIN		
ARTHRITIS, GOUT AND SUB-ACUTE GOUT		
PMS/MOOD SWINGS DUE TO SEROTONIN FLUCTUATIONS		
TOTAL SCORE		

CHAPTER 6

Tracking Your Blood Sugars

This is the most important lesson, as excess sugar can cause yeast infections, heart diseases, weight gain, and diabetes. It is very important that you have the discipline to measure the blood glucose in the blood before you eat and one hour after you have eaten so that you can really work out which carb is causing that negative reaction.

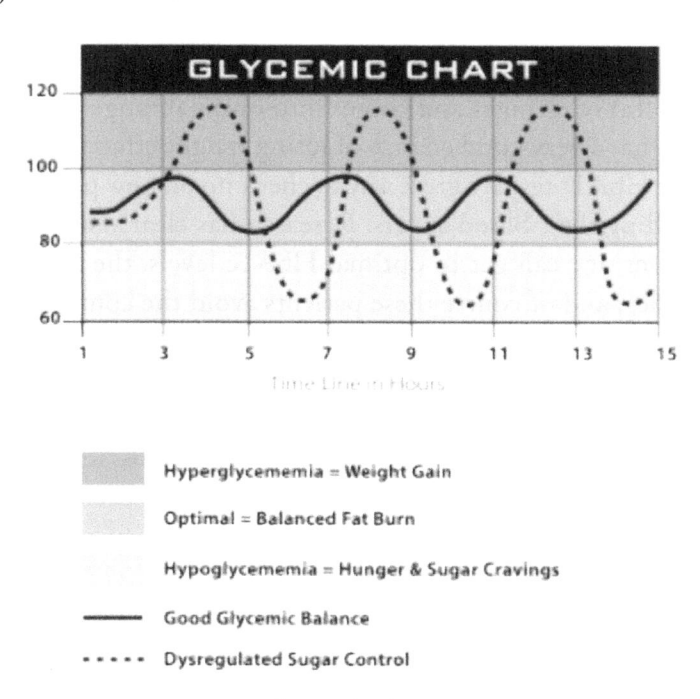

Glycemic chart.

If you look at the preceding chart, the dashed line is the result of a high-GI food. The blood sugar will rise sharply, causing weight gain that is soon followed by a crash that induces hunger and sugar cravings. This is a classic pattern that erodes the leptin sensitivity of the body.

Testing Stability with Hemoglobin A1c (HbA1c)

The red blood cell has a life span of about four months or 120 days. And glucose combines with hemoglobin to form a substance called glycohemoglobin. The quantity of glycohemoglobin formed is in direct proportion to the amount of glucose within the blood during that 120-day life span. This process is called glycosylation.

If the patient has had too many sugars during that timeline, the amount of HbA1c increases and is irreversible. In summary, if the blood glucose level is consistently elevated, then the patient's ability to recover from diabetes and obesity is poor. However, if the HbA1c changes and comes into optimal ranges, then the patient has a very good chance of losing weight effectively.

The HbA1c test is a great way to check up on how patients are controlling their blood sugars. Research has clearly shown that the closer one can get to optimal HbA1c levels, the better the outcomes; and of course these patients avoid the complications associated with diabetes and obesity.

Fasting blood-glucose levels are also very important, as these will express how well the individual is doing on a daily basis. Steady effort in the right direction will pay huge weight-loss rewards and ultimately improve the life and longevity of the patient.

GLUCOSE TEST	CONVENTIONAL RANGE	OPTIMAL RANGE
Hba1c	< 7%	4.1 - 5.5%
BLOOD GLUCOSE	65 - 115 mg/dl	80-90 mg/dl

Chapter 7

Testing for Estrogen Dominance

Natural estrogen is an important hormone to humans, particularly for female reproduction, and it works in conjunction with the hormone progesterone to create human female fertility. In women, estrogen's opposing hormone is called progesterone. In men, estrogen's opposing hormone is called testosterone.

These days, many people often suffer high levels of estrogens within their bodies. When the levels go too high or progesterone and testosterone levels go too low, we call it "estrogen dominance." This is more frequently seen in women, but men can suffer from it too. The usual symptoms are mood changes, sugar cravings, weight gain, fatigue, sleep problems, menstrual changes, lowered sex drive, fluid retention, and breast enlargement. Many women only report having one or two symptoms, but others could recognize all. Estrogen dominance is at its worst during the perimenopausal and menopausal years, but I have seen women of all ages suffering from it.

Female Questions

Did you experience a premature puberty or early breast development?

- Estrogen encourages breast growth and maturation of the reproductive organs in girls. Young girls are now starting puberty much earlier than they did in the recent past. Two generations ago, young girls had their first period around

age fourteen. Presently, many girls experience their first menstruation around age nine to twelve.
- The greater the young girl's exposure to high levels of estrogen throughout her lifetime, the greater her risk of succumbing to hormonal-related disorders in later life.
- Initially, adult women may experience estrogen dominance as cyclical migraine headaches, irregular menstrual periods, weight gain from water retention, anxiety and irritability, and sore, swollen breasts.

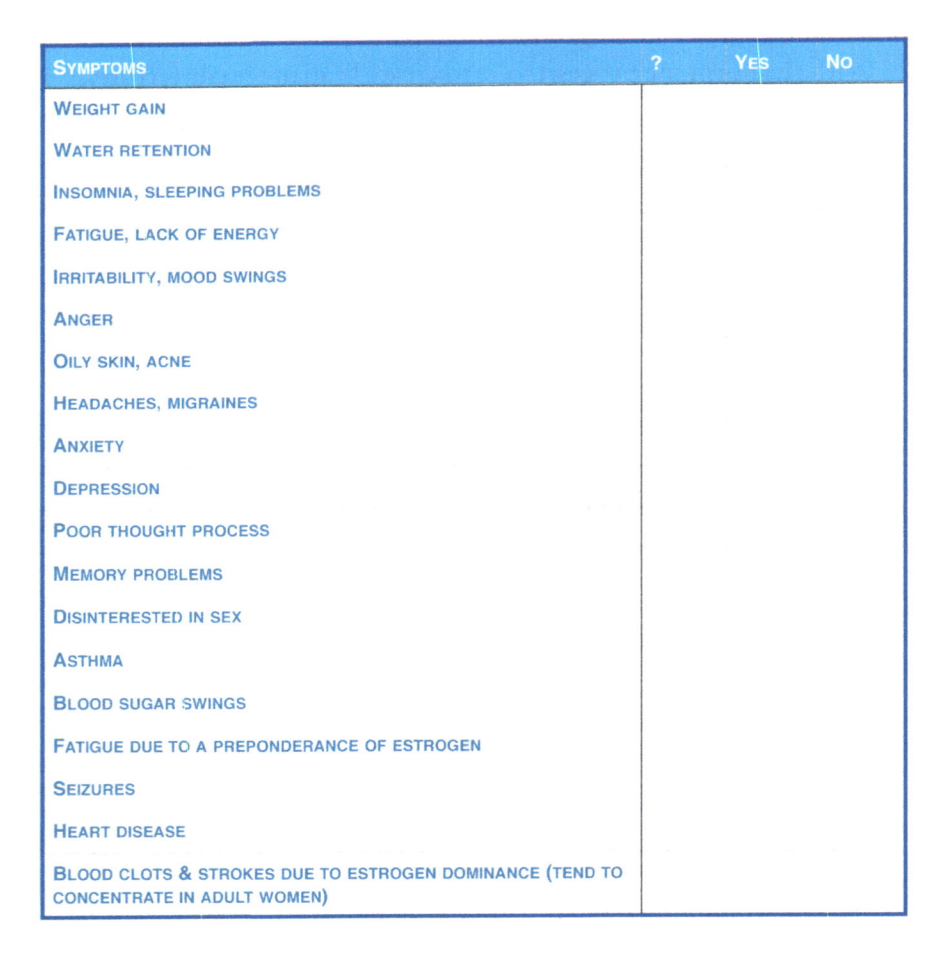

Symptoms	?	Yes	No
Weight gain			
Water retention			
Insomnia, sleeping problems			
Fatigue, lack of energy			
Irritability, mood swings			
Anger			
Oily skin, acne			
Headaches, migraines			
Anxiety			
Depression			
Poor thought process			
Memory problems			
Disinterested in sex			
Asthma			
Blood sugar swings			
Fatigue due to a preponderance of estrogen			
Seizures			
Heart disease			
Blood clots & strokes due to estrogen dominance (tend to concentrate in adult women)			

Male Questions

- Young boys may experience estrogen dominance as tardy puberty. Estrogen opposes the effects of testosterone. Estrogen-dominant young boys and teens will experience a decreased level of masculine development. In hypogonadal boys, where testosterone development is deficient, estrogen dominance can result in breast development in boys, a condition called gynecomastia (often referred to as "man boobs").
- Did you experience a delayed puberty or some element of male boobs? Do you find it hard to build muscle?

Both Men and Women can Experience:

Allergies and nasal congestion are worsened by estrogen dominance. Prescription drugs used to treat them also induce greater levels of estrogen dominance.

A few scientists and doctors attribute autoimmune diseases[1] like lupus and Sjögren's syndrome to hormonal imbalance[2]. Estrogen must be balanced by another hormone called progesterone. Therefore, if a woman is prescribed estrogens long-term in the form of birth-control pills or hormone-replacement therapy, or eats far too many types of meat laced with estrogen derivatives, the estrogen levels will start to rise and become out of balance compared to the progesterone. This situation is called estrogen dominance. Following is a table that shows the optimal ranges required for good health.

---

1   Ilia J. Elenkov and George P. Chrousos, "Stress Hormones, Th1/Th2 patterns, Pro/Anti-inflammatory Cytokines and Susceptibility to Disease," *Trends in Endocrinology & Metabolism* 10(9) (1999): 359–368.

2   S. Ansar Ahmed, W. J. Penhale, and N. Talal, "Sex hormones, immune responses, and autoimmune diseases. Mechanisms of sex hormone action," *American Journal of Pathology* 121(3) (1985): 531–551.

Table to Show Optimal Ranges for Estrogen and Progesterone

Hormone blood test	Conventional Range	Optimal Range	Abnormal Range
Estradiol - women *	0 -528 pg/ml	352 - 528	0 - 351
Progesterone - women *	3 - 27 ng/ml	13-23	0 -10
Estradiol - men	10 - 56 pg/ml	10-25	High > 30
Progesterone - men	0.1 - 1.3 ng/ml	1.0 - 1.2	0 - 0.9

The twenty-first day is the best day to test premenopausal (for pregnancy) women and any day for a postmenopausal woman. Estrogen levels should be measured against progesterone to see if they are in balance with each other. Men can test their progesterone levels at any time, preferably in the morning.

Chapter 8

Testing for Progesterone Deficiency

Estrogen must be balanced by the body's hormone called progesterone. Progesterone is the opposite hormone to estrogen, and levels must remain in balance with each other; otherwise illness will ensue.

Therefore, if a woman is prescribed estrogens long-term in the form of birth-control pills or hormone-replacement therapy, or eats far too much meat laced with estrogen derivatives, estrogen levels will start to rise and become out of balance compared to progesterone. If a man consumes too much alcohol, fast foods, excess coffee, the estrogen will start to rise. This situation is called estrogen dominance.

The chart on the following page shows the symptoms of progesterone deficiency.

KEY: If you scored greater than four "yes" answers, it is likely you have a progesterone deficiency. Get your levels tested and start following progesterone-boosting therapy.

Symptoms	?	Yes	No
Swollen breasts			
Headaches/Migraines			
Anxiety			
Irregular menses			
Cramping/fibroids			
Infertility			
Spotting before period			
Bloating & Gas			
Acne			
Weight gain			
Low libido			
Mood swings			
Depression			
PMS			
Fuzzy thinking			
Joint pain			
Breast Cancer			

Chapter 9

Testing for Testosterone Deficiency

As with all the hormones, testosterone declines with age, and men and women older than thirty will have a certain degree of deficiency, namely because DHEA levels decline after the age of twenty-five to thirty years. DHEA converts into the androgen strength and sexuality hormone called testosterone.

Commonly thought of as a male hormone, testosterone is required by both the sexes, as it relates to muscle development and libidinal function.

Testosterone is an anabolic hormone that builds muscle[1] and reduces fat[2] and that can be easily tested using a simple blood test.

On the following page is a table that shows the symptoms of testosterone deficiency.

KEY: If you scored greater than four "yes" answers, it is likely you have a testosterone deficiency. Get your levels tested and start following testosterone-boosting therapy or start a course of bioidentical testosterone cream.

---

[1] Fred R. Sattler, Carmen Castaneda-Sceppa, Ellen F. Binder, E. Todd Schroeder, Ying Wang, Shalender Bhasin, Miwa Kawakubo, Yolanda Stewart, Kevin E. Yarasheski, Jagadish Ulloor, Patrick Colletti, Ronenn Roubenoff, and Stanley P. Azen, "Testosterone and Growth Hormone Improve Body Composition and Muscle Performance in Older Men," *JCEM* 94 (2009): 1991–2001.

[2] Shalender Bhasin, Thomas W. Storer, Nancy Berman, Kevin E. Yarasheski, Brenda Clevenger, Jeffrey Phillips, W. Paul Lee, Thomas J. Bunnell, and Richard Casaburi, "Testosterone Replacement Increases Fat-Free Mass and Muscle Size in Hypogonadal Men," *JCEM* 82 (1997): 407–413.

Symptoms	?	Yes	No
Decline in general health			
Joint pain, myalgia			
Excessive sweating			
Need for more sleep			
Fatigue			
Nervous, restless			
Spotting before period			
Anxiety			
Physical exhaustion			
Decreased muscle size			
Decreased strength			
Decreased morning erections			
Decreased libido			
Decreased levels of sexual pleasure			
Decreased facial hair			

Total Blood Testosterone	Conventional Range	Optimal Range	Deficient Range
Male	10 - 35 nmol/L 3000 - 10000 pg/ml 3000 - 1000 ng/dL	24 7000 700	0 -19 0 - 5500 0 - 550
Female	0.3 - 1.7 nmol/L 100 - 500 pg/ml 10 - 50 ng/ml	1.2 350 35	0 - 0.9 0 - 250 0 - 25
Free Testosterone			
Male	6 - 26.5 pg/ml	20 - 26 pg/ml	0 - 15

Testosterone levels decline gradually with age in human beings; this is clear from the previous table. The clinical significance of this decrease is debated. There is disagreement about when to treat aging men with testosterone-replacement therapy.

N.B: Testosterone therapy warrants the advice and management of a competent physician. Measuring free testosterone in the blood is also important, as it represents a true picture of how much testosterone is available for use by the body.

In men the optimal range for free testosterone is 20–26 pg/ml[3]. Unfortunately, the average lab or MD will use a range of 6–26.5 pg/ml. This allows men to get unnecessarily ill, as the reference range is so wide that it's hard to spot the connections between disease development and testosterone decline[4]. A low level of testosterone places every man at greater risk for virtually every age-related disease. Following is a table to show the blood testosterone decline over the years[5].

MALE/AGE GROUPS	MEAN
30 - 39	12.84
40 - 49	12.42
50 - 59	11.38
60 -69	10.71
70 - PLUS	9.5

---

3   W. Faloon, "MD Physician's guide: Using blood tests to safely induce weight loss," *Life Extension* 15(6) (2009): 42–63.

4   S. Turhan, C. Tulunay, S. Güleç, et al, "The association between androgen levels and pre- mature coronary artery disease in men," *Coronary Artery Dissease* 18(3) (2007): 159–162.

5   http://www.lef.org/magazine/mag2010/jun2010_Startling-Low-Testosterone-Blood-Levels-in-Male-Life-Extension-Members_01.htm

The American Society of Andrology's position is[6]: "Testosterone replacement therapy in aging men is indicated when both clinical symptoms and signs suggestive of androgen deficiency and decreased Testosterone levels are present."

The American Association of Clinical Endocrinologists says: "Hypogonadism is defined as a free Testosterone level that is below the lower limit of normal for young adult control subjects. Previously, age-related decreases in free Testosterone were once accepted as normal. Currently, they are not considered normal. Patients with low-normal to subnormal range Testosterone levels warrant a clinical trial of Testosterone.

Using salivary measurements, the optimal ranges are as follows:

Salivary Testosterone	Conventional Range	Optimal Range	Deficient Range
Morning	290 - 520 pmol/L	420	0 - 300
Mid-Day	190 - 350 pmol/L	300	0 - 240
Afternoon	140 - 220 pmol/L	200	0 - 170
Evening	50 - 160 pmol/L	100	0 - 100

On the following page is an example of a patient's recorded testosterone levels at the four points throughout the day.

As you can see from the salivary testosterone numbers, this patient is clearly in a low testosterone pattern. We should all be aiming for the optimal range at all points throughout the day.

It took me personally about six months to raise my free testosterone from 9.26 to 23.48. Testosterone therapy takes time to see results. Most results take about three months to see roughly 30–40 percent improvements. I lost approximately twenty-two pounds of fat and gained ten pounds of muscle.

Remember, there are strong connections between low testosterone and the development of diabetes, heart disease, and reduced

---

6   "Testosterone replacement therapy for male aging: ASA position statement," *Journal of Androl* 27(2) (2006): 133–134.

life span. Monitor to see how the numbers change every three months until you are in the optimal range.

N.B: Low-dose testosterone therapy to achieve optimal health and resist disease is not the same as bodybuilding. Bodybuilders take in one month what it would take to treat a low-testosterone male for three to four years. We are looking for optimal health, not an extreme muscular physique.

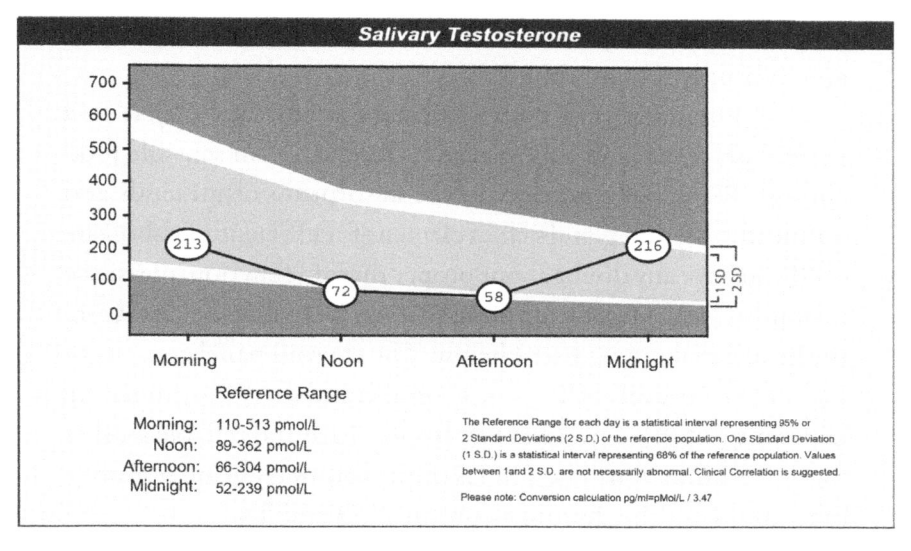

Salivary Testosterone

Morning: 213
Noon: 72
Afternoon: 58
Midnight: 216

Reference Range
Morning: 110-513 pmol/L
Noon: 89-362 pmol/L
Afternoon: 66-304 pmol/L
Midnight: 52-239 pmol/L

The Reference Range for each day is a statistical interval representing 95% or 2 Standard Deviations (2 S.D.) of the reference population. One Standard Deviation (1 S.D.) is a statistical interval representing 68% of the reference population. Values between 1 and 2 S.D. are not necessarily abnormal. Clinical Correlation is suggested.

Please note: Conversion calculation pg/ml=pMol/L / 3.47

Sample of Salivary Testosterone Test showing hypogonadism.

CHAPTER 10

Testing the Thyroid Gland

For proper thyroid function, you need a daily source of clean iodine, such as seaweed supplements or kelp or even a trace-mineral supplement. The thyroid is able to pick up iodine via the stomach and liver only if your pH is perfect.

Pure human energy comes through when the body is in a perfect pH zone, and this in turn is dependent on sensible food choices. Perfect pH maximizes the absorption of minerals and iodine, the thyroid gland's chief element for efficient metabolism.

If you have any doubt about proper thyroid function, please see your physician. Also, please observe how close your test results are to the optimal ranges listed below. The thyroid panel consists of looking at the levels of T3, T4, T uptake, and thyroid-stimulating hormone (TSH). The TSH test is a sensitive and reliable marker for thyroid function. The TSH is the key pituitary gland hormone that stimulates the thyroid to produce T3 and T4.

A TSH level shows the level of communication between the pituitary and thyroid and the level of stimulation it's receiving. These are important hormones in getting the body its full energy quotient.

	STANDARD US UNITS	STANDARD INT'L UNITS	OPTIMAL RANGE	ALARM RANGE
TSH	0.9 - 3.0 uIU/ml	0.9 - 3.0 mIU/L	1.3 - 2.0 uIU/ml 1.3 - 2.0 milli U/L	< 0.3 uIU/ml > 4.0 mIU/L

Medical doctors, in order to identify thyroid pathology in their patients, typically use the standard reference ranges for TSH, which as you can tell are very wide and therefore slightly insensitive for testing subclinical conditions of the thyroid before it becomes diseased. Most of the time the conventional physician will not be able to diagnose a subclinical disorder.

However, the optimal ranges are far more helpful in diagnosing a subclinical thyroid disorder. Functional thyroid disorders should be evaluated against the optimal ranges.

The thyroid is also vulnerable to autoimmune diseases, such as Graves' disease and Hashimoto's disease. In functional medicine, we understand that most autoimmune diseases come from a leaky gut paired with burnt-out adrenal glands.

Measure your thyroid

Your body temperature = your metabolic heat

The hormones secreted by the thyroid and, to a lesser degree, the adrenal glands largely control your metabolism. Although blood hormone testing for adrenals and thyroid are common, there is considerable evidence that the current tests for the diagnosis of hypothyroidism (low thyroid function) are not sensitive enough.

With adrenal function taken into consideration, the role of the thyroid gland can be assessed by basically measuring your body temperature. All you need is a digital thermometer.

Instructions:

1. Use only a *digital* thermometer, not mercury or an ear thermometer.
2. Please measure your temperature orally and place the thermometer deep under your tongue. Do not take your temperature from your underarm or ear.
3. Take only one reading each day, and record history.
4. Take your first morning temperature approximately one to three minutes *after* waking up; have the thermometer by the bedside table for easy reach.

5. Approximate body temperature should be 98.0–98.6 degrees F (37 degrees C); if yours is less than 98.0, consider doing a thyroid function test (blood) and iodine patch test.
6. Monitor daily and see if the body temperature starts to rise back to optimal with thyroid support vitamins and daily iodine support.

Measure Your Iodine

The iodine patch test is also excellent for assessing an iodine deficiency. This essential element is absolutely necessary for proper thyroid function, yet many people in the world suffer from an iodine deficiency. Other similar elements such as chlorine, bromine, and fluoride can deplete iodine, and they are abundant in our toxic environment. Iodine deficiency is a major cause of hypothyroidism, obesity, low energy, constipation, and weakened immunity.

Instructions:
1. Using an ear cleaner, dip into the 3 percent iodine solution and paint a three-centimeter square patch of iodine above the elbow (as hands and wrists are washed during the course of a human day). Allow it to dry.
2. Record the time you made the patch.
3. Avoid washing the area for at least twenty-four hours.
4. Note the time that the iodine patch fades out.

Interpretation of Fading Time

< 8 hours = serious iodine deficiency/get tested for hypothyroidism

> 8 hours = moderate iodine deficiency/get tested for hypothyroidism

< 24 hours = mild iodine deficiency/eat more iodine-containing foods

> 24 hours = iodine reserves are good

Please fill out this table so you know which gland needs attending to. Be sure to choose only one answer. If the answer doesn't apply, leave the box blank.

Signs & Symptoms	✓	Thyroid	✓	Adrenal
Body type		Overweight global		Pot belly
Skin		Oily/greasy		Dry & thin
Stress		Okay		Poor resistance to stress
Mood		Depression		Anxiety
Blood Sugar		Normal to high		Hypoglycemic
Blood Pressure		Slightly higher		Low blood pressure
Ligaments		Inflexibility		Prone to aches & strains
Prone to cold hands & feet		No		Yes
Perspiration		More oily than sweaty		Excessive or history of
Puffy eyes vs Dark circles		Puffy bags under eyes		Tendency to dark circles
Weight Gain		Difficulty losing weight		Difficulty gaining weight
Water Retention		Usual		Tendency to be dry
		Total Score		Total Score

Count up how many you scored in each.
How did you score?
Is your thyroid slower or is it your adrenals?
Are both running as slow as each other?
Burning fat is dependent on having two key organs working well, and these are the thyroid and adrenal glands. Using this information, you can now emphasize either adrenal or thyroid

by supporting them through supplements and natural hormones and eating according to your metabolic type.

To "burn fat" well, you need to understand what your metabolism is doing and choose the appropriate *food ratios* of protein and fats vs. carbohydrates to match your current metabolism. Through metabolic typing, you can start to modify the way your hormones work for the better.

CHAPTER 11

Testing Your Leptin, Adiponectin, Ghrelin, and Melatonin Levels

You will be able to answer most of these questions from previous self-assessments, and some will require some information from your MD/osteopath/naturopath/chiropractor local labs.

Biochemical Clues

1. What is your blood sugar after twelve hours of fasting? If it is greater than 92.5mg/dl, this indicates leptin resistance (LR).
2. Take an HbA1c test. Having a result > 5.6 percent indicates LR.
3. Measure your CRP. This is a measurement for inflammation in the body, which is a sign of LR. It ideally should be below 1.0mg/L.
4. Check your cholesterol and triglycerides. Having high levels of both is a sure sign that leptin signaling is damaged.
5. Men—measure your testosterone, for levels too low indicate LR.
6. Women—measure for high DHEA and low progesterone, as these indicate LR.
7. Measure your thyroid-stimulating hormone (TSH). Low levels indicate hypothyroidism and LR.

Physical Clues

1. Body fat percentage—if you are male and have a body fat percentage > 20 percent, then LR has started. Each 5 percent

more increases the severity of LR, making weight loss near impossible without some leptin hormone correction.

2. Higher blood pressure—blood pressure > 130/90 indicates LR.
3. Less than seven hours of undisturbed sleep indicates LR.
4. Ultrasound, CT, or MRI of the liver and pancreas are also important clues, as the imaging techniques will show fatty deposits around the abdominal organs in both men and women.
5. Fibroids and ovarian cysts are indicative of LR in females.

If you connect the dots, you will understand that leptin is a key player in making or breaking your weight-loss process. All the hormones are interrelated. One needs to juggle all eight in harmony to achieve an amazing fat-blasting program.

Measuring Your Adiponectin Levels—This blood test needs to be processed and interpreted by your local physician, MD, or DO. There is an excellent test from Genova Diagnostics that can measure this hormone in conjunction with insulin function. The test is used as an assessment of the risk for diabetes and metabolic syndrome.

Measuring Ghrelin—Recently test kits are being produced that can measure ghrelin. However, this hunger hormone can be kept in check by making sure the leptin and adiponectin pathways are functioning correctly, meals are on time, and that allergy and parasite stress are zero.

Measuring Melatonin—This can be done using a simple saliva test that measures the amount of melatonin. The test should be taken around 10:00 PM so as to ascertain the amount of melatonin being produced and to see if it is sufficient to allow for sleep induction and sleep maintenance. It can be measured at BioHealth labs, USA, while measuring the adrenal and sex-hormone stress profile (205V).

:::
THE SOLUTION
:::

Chapter 12

Controlling Your Eight Fat-Causing Hormones

Our Natural Steroids

Our bodies' complete and healthy functioning relies on having adequate amounts of natural steroids activating and balancing our metabolism, mood, digestion, and detoxification.

Cholesterol, the basic raw material of all hormones, converts into the first hormone called Pregnenolone in the adrenal glands with the help of the healthy liver enzymes. Pregnenolone kicks off an amazing cascade of life-giving hormones, and when healthy the production is balanced.

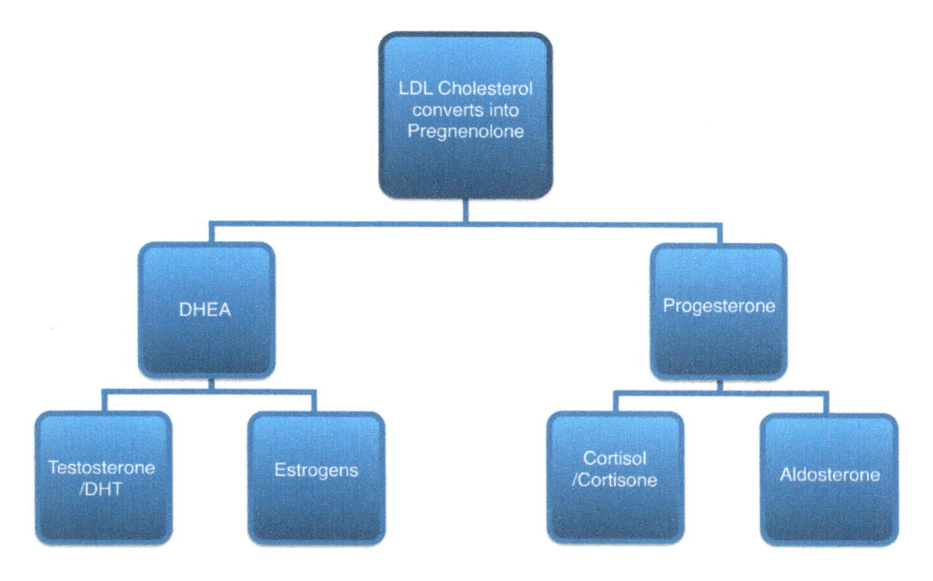

The normal steroid pathway.

THE TOTAL FAT CURE

> **KEY POINT:** When people become overstressed, the hormone pathway changes for the worse and looks more like the following figure, whereby Pregnenolone and Progesterone are entirely converted into cortisol. This is called the Pregnenolone/cortisol steal, and cause the decline of DHEA levels.

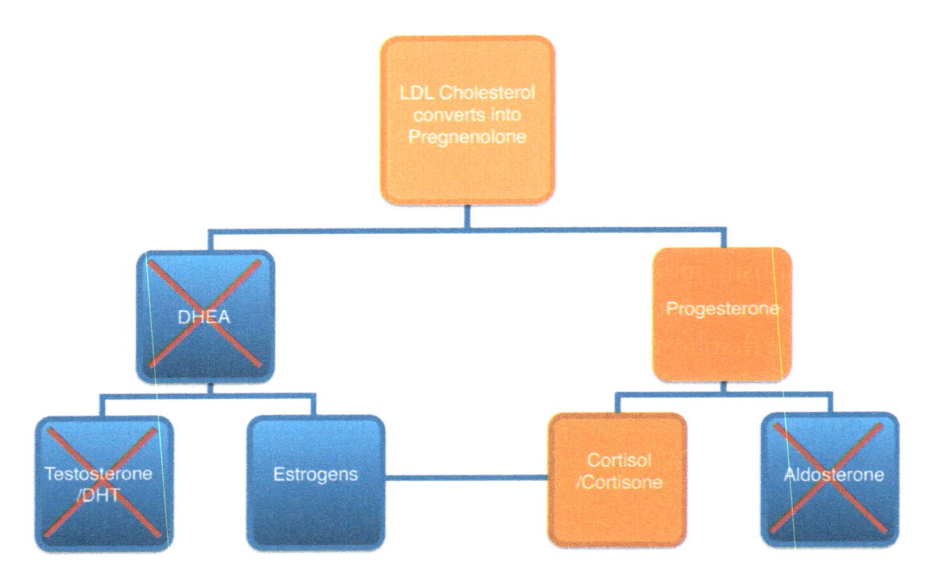

```
                LDL Cholesterol
                converts into
                Pregnenolone
               /              \
           DHEA (X)         Progesterone
          /      \          /          \
    Testosterone  Estrogens  Cortisol   Aldosterone (X)
       /DHT (X)              /Cortisone
```

The stressed steroid pathway.

In the next couple of pages, you will find out how to control those hormones that have gone out of balance. Applying this key action starts to create the right hormone levels. Once the energy levels pick up, use that energy to create a good lifestyle.

How to Balance Cortisol

Practice meditation, learn yoga, and take the right amount of natural hormones to complement your glandular function.

- How did you score on your adrenal tests/ questionnaires? (see Chapter 5)
- Can you reduce your stress by changing your lifestyle?
- Do you think you should test for food allergies or parasites?

Adrenal Results and Suggested Therapy

- **If you scored high cortisol levels** = use one or two Seriphos capsules four to six hours before a spike in Cortisol (usually experienced as anxiety or panic), to lower the levels and use DHEA 25mg/meditate/do yoga/walk/relax. *Seriphos will lower abnormally high cortisol levels.*
- **If you scored low cortisol levels** = use Pregnenolone, thirty to forty-five drops/day and licorice/low-dose cortisone to increase the levels and use low-dose DHEA 3mg–6mg/day/rest/a little strength training 2 week/ meditate/ yoga. Never use Seriphos. Cortico B5 and B6, Vit. C daily and an adrenal glandular.

Mentally and Physically Rebuilding the Adrenals

There are three key ways of positively influencing both mind and body on this program:

1. Meditation
2. Yoga or tai chi or chi gong
3. Natural hormones

1. How to Meditate Simply

Several patients over the years have asked me to tell them a recipe for good meditation, and in my more than two decades of practicing meditation, I have given them some simple ideas that helped them to recover[1] from illness[2]. I will share them with you now.

---

[1] Christopher R.K. MacLean, Kenneth G. Walton, Stig R. Wenneberg, Debra K. Levitsky, Joseph P. Mandarino, Rafiq Waziri, Stephen L. Hillis, and Robert H. Schneider, "Effects of the transcendental meditation program on adaptive mechanisms: Changes in hormone levels and responses to stress after 4 months of practice," *Psychoneuroendocrinology* 22 (4) (1997): 277–295.

[2] Linda E Carlson, Michael Speca, Kamala D. Patel, and Eileen Goodey, "Mindfulness-based

4. Find a quiet place that is free from any loud noises (I sometimes use earplugs to achieve this).

5. Get into a comfortable posture, by either sitting in a chair with a straight back or, more traditionally, sitting cross-legged on a cushion on the floor.

6. Take a moment or two to install a relaxed mind by allowing your body to settle. Think about gratitude and thank your version of spirituality for everything good in your world now, and be really sincere. Your god knows when you are lying and when you are being genuine.

7. As you become more relaxed, focus on the gentle movements of the breath in and out of the chest.

8. As you breathe in through the nose, and count silently within your mind, "One, two, three, four, five,", then hold the breath for a further four seconds, and then release for five seconds gently out through the mouth.

9. During the breathing cycles, focus on your goals (becoming slimmer, fitter, and healthier). Imagine eating healthy foods and exercising, while allowing the harmony of the thoughts and the harmony of the breath to meld with each other. Become one in the moment. Serotonin starts to build up at this point due to the happy images and the balanced breathing.

10. Practice this cycle of breathing meditation for approximately ten to fifteen minutes per day. Practice twice a day if you can, in the morning first thing and as the last thing before retiring to bed.

11. As you become more proficient in it, then extend the time to about twenty to thirty minutes as is comfortable. Be comfortable in your time.

---

stress reduction in relation to quality of life, mood, symptoms of stress and levels of Cortisol, Dehydroepiandrosterone sulfate (DHEAS) and Melatonin in breast and prostate cancer out- patients," *Psychoneuroendocrinology* 29 (4) (2004): 448–474.

Practice meditation as you wake up first thing in the morning and as the last thing at night before sleeping. If you do not want to meditate to control your stress levels, then consider regular massage as a passive activity to induce great levels of relaxation, or consider simple yoga.

2. Cool Down with Yoga

Yoga is a great way to relax the muscles from an intense workout. Keeping your muscles stretched out post-workout helps repair muscles faster and makes them stronger. As your muscles get stronger, you are regaining your youth!

Try doing yoga stretches (three sun salutations, breathing cycles indicated):

1. While standing, stretch up to the sky with your arms (breathe in).

2. Then swoop down with your arms and touch your toes, like a hamstring stretch (breathe out).

3. Leave your palms on the ground and stretch one leg all the way back behind you so that the toes are touching the ground (breathe in).

4. While keeping the palms on the ground, stretch your other leg to join the first leg. It looks like a push-up with straight arms (breathe out).

5. In the same push-up position, make a bridge with your body (breathe in).

6. In the same push-up position, again with straight arms, get your chin and chest to touch the floor while leaving your backside in the air, then flatten out your whole body on the floor while keeping your hands by your shoulders (breathe out).

7. Go into a cobra position; lying flat, push up from your arms (breathe in). Arch your entire back with only straight arms and enjoy the extension. Lean your head and neck also in extension, open your mouth, and stick your tongue out as far as you can and hold for a few seconds, then close your mouth (breathe in and out).

8. Go back into the push-up position and with arms extended, bring one leg up next to your hands while leaving the other leg in a stretched position (breathe in).

9. Now place both feet up by your hands. You should be back into a bilateral hamstring stretch, palms on the floor (breathe out).

10. Now stretch up to the sky with your arms (breathe in).

11. Drink some water and give thanks to life, love, and health.

3. Natural Hormones

There are two key hormones that help to rebalance the adrenal glands themselves, and the amount and ratio is dictated by the stage of burnout that one is in. These are Pregnenolone and DHEA, and they can be harvested from Mexican yams.

Pregnenolone

Pregnenolone and DHEA show profound anti-cortisol (stress hormone) activity and can be an accurate measurement of how well you cope with stress.

Less stress can mean a longer life. If you're stressed, you need to create a new lifestyle, improve your diet, and use natural hormones to rejuvenate your body and mind. The reward will be longevity and peace.

Pregnenolone is the foundation for all hormones in the human body. Cholesterol is turned into Pregnenolone, which is then converted into other hormones, such as DHEA and progesterone. Pregnenolone is one of the key molecules used in the body's resistance against stress, and the brain actively uses it for memory function too.

It is produced in large amounts when we are young, and after the age of thirty our production of this precious substance starts to wane and declines slowly over time until we get to seventy. Later in life we produce a tenth of the amount we produced when in our teens and twenties.

It is a very effective pro-hormone, and as such I prescribe it in low doses to my patients who are suffering from adrenal fatigue, exhaustion or burnout, memory disorders, low mood, and depression.

❱ **KEY POINT: Without Pregnenolone, there is no human life, as it makes all the important life-giving hormones.**

❱ **TESTING: You can tell how much Pregnenolone is in your system because it directly relates to the total production of DHEA and progesterone.**

Low progesterone and DHEA levels indicate low Pregnenolone, especially if the patient suffers from high cholesterol. High cholesterol fails to convert into the usable Pregnenolone in the liver and adrenals.

Therapeutic Dose:
Many of my adrenal fatigued/burnt-out patients take Pregnenolone in small amounts, 1-18mg in three divided doses throughout the day to assist in the production of both progesterone and DHEA (when you wake up, at noon, and in the afternoon, about 5:00 PM). The stage of burnout that you are "in" determines the dose of yam Pregnenolone needed to replace the missing production of your own hormones.

- Stage 1 = 6–8 drops 3 x day
- Stage 2 = 9–12 drops 3 x day

- Stage 3 = 12–18 drops 3 x day

The above dosages are based on my training and research in Functional Medicine. Liquid Pregnenolone is far better than the capsule or tablet versions, as it absorbs almost completely through the gums and tongue. The capsule or tablet versions experience stomach acids, and the acids reduce their potency. Cream-based Pregnenolone is also acceptable as long as different areas of skin are used to avoid oversaturation of Pregnenolone in one area.

Side effects of excess Pregnenolone can be acne, greasy hair and skin, and headaches. Simply lower the dosage if you experience any of these.

DHEA: The Fountain of Youth

DHEA is another important hormone. Pregnenolone and DHEA levels must be adequate, otherwise we cannot cope with stress or aging. Pregnenolone and DHEA show profound anti-cortisol activity[3] and as such can be an accurate measurement of how well you cope with stress. Some of the diseases associated with low levels of DHEA in both men and women are cardiovascular diseases[4], Alzheimer's disease, depression, sleep disorders, weight gain or obesity, diabetes, hypothyroidism, lupus, and cancer.

DHEA goes on to make the hormones testosterone and estrogen. DHEA is cortisol's nemesis because it has anti-obesity effects by reducing fat-cell stimulation and excess insulin and smothering hunger.

---

3   G. Pincus, H. Hoagland, C. H. Wilson, and N. J. Fay, "Effects on industrial production of the administration of 3 Pregnenolone to factory workers," II. *Psychosomatic Medicine* 7 (1945): 347–352.

4   H. Kawano, H. Yasue, A. Kitagawa, et al, "Dehydroepiandrosterone supplementation improves endothelial function and Insulin sensitivity in men," *J Clinical Endocrinoogyl & Metabolism* 88 (2003): 3190–3195

DHEA rises with age and peaks around twenty-five to thirty in humans, after which it steadily declines. By the time we're seventy-five years of age, our DHEA levels have reduced to about 15–20 percent of what they were at twenty years of age.

Too little DHEA will cause several diseases directly related to its deficiency. Because DHEA is a key building block of estrogen and testosterone, it has an enormous effect on thyroid function and allows the conversion of T4 into the more active thyroid hormone called T3[5].

	CONVENTIONAL RANGE	OPTIMAL RANGE	DEFICIENT RANGE
MALES	0.7 - 21.2 umol/L	11.0 - 18	0 - 6.90
FEMALES	2.8 - 16.6 umol/L	9.0 - 12	0 - 6.90

Therapeutic Dose

The easiest way to treat DHEA deficiencies is to go the oral route. You will want the expert advice of a physician when rebalancing your hormones, as underdosing and overdosing have their consequences. Here are some guidelines for therapy.

- **Women:** 1–10mg/day 1 x day
- **Men:** 1–15mg/day 1 x day

N.B Caution with DHEA, as it is *very* potent. Side effects of excess DHEA are acne, greasy skin, facial hair growth, and headaches. If you are prone to greasy skin, avoid using DHEA in large amounts, only use 1mg/day, and slowly increase the dose until one notices the greasiness of the skin or spots, then remember the tipping-point dose and remain under it.

---

[5] J. L. Foldes et al, "Dehydroepiandrosterone sulfate (DS), Dehydroepiandrosterone (D) and "free" Dehydroepiandrosterone (FD) in the plasma with thyroid diseases," *Horm Metab Res* 15 (1983): 623–624.

❯ **KEY POINT: Clinical studies noted a Western diet such as the Standard American Diet (SAD diet) had the effect of lowering the DHEA levels.**

Once again consuming allergic foods causes an increase in cortisol, which in turn reduces the levels of DHEA. DHEA studies as related to the development of cancer have shown that those patients with low levels of DHEA have greater risks of prostate cancer, gastric[6] cancer, bladder cancer[7], and lung cancer[8].

In conclusion, it is important to have levels of DHEA accurately tested and monitored because the risks of developing age-related, degenerative disease are directly proportional to the amount of DHEA you have in your body.

Maladaptation to stress causes the DHEA/cortisol ratios to shift in a negative direction. Balance is the key, and both DHEA and cortisol are needed by the body in order to age well.

How to Balance Insulin

Balancing your cortisol levels and having regular balanced meals and proper bedtimes achieve this. Follow a low-GI diet. There's a good guide later in the book called **Glycemic Index of Selected Foods**. It's easy to follow.

Reducing stress, getting rid of chronic gut infections, and removing all allergies from the diet creates great sugar-balancing

---

[6] G. B. Gordon, K. J. Helzlsouer, A. J. Alberg, and G. W. Comstock, "Serum levels of Dehydroepiandrosterone and Dehydroepiandrosterone sulfate and the risk of developing gastric cancer," *Cancer Epidemiology Biomarkers & Prevention* (1993): 2.

[7] G. B. Gordon, K. J. Helzlsouer, and G. W. Comstock, "Serum levels of Dehydroepiandrosterone and its sulfate and the risk of developing bladder cancer," *Cancer Res 51*(5) (1991): 1366–1369.

[8] J. M. Bhatavdekar, D. D. Patel, P. R. Chikhlikar, R. H. Mehta, H. H. Vora, N. H. Karelia, et al, "Levels of circulating peptide and steroid hormones in men with lung cancer," *Neoplasma* 41(2) (1994): 101–103.

effects. Also, two herbs called Goat's Rue extract and Gymnema Sylvestre are excellent at lowering blood sugar. For more information, please see my book *Curing Diabetes in Seven Steps*, as these two key herbs are instrumental in changing the blood sugar levels naturally.

How to Balance Estrogen

Relief is found in detoxing the body from estrogens by eating cruciferous vegetables (broccoli, cabbage, brussels sprouts), ramping up the liver function (milk thistle), and making sure that the blood-chemistry liver enzymes (zinc and selenium) are within optimal ranges or as close as possible.

Hormonally, progesterone therapy for both men and women under thirty years of age will also achieve great results by making up the deficient hormone and rebooting the endocrine system and the organs of the body. Only a physician trained in bioidentical hormone-replacement therapy (BHRT) can administer progesterone and estrogen therapy. It takes an element of accuracy and retesting levels.

Prescriptions for BHRT in the form of oral tablets, sublinguals, or transdermal creams are the normal method of absorption.

Calcium D-Glucarate: The Natural Anti-Estrogen FAT BURNER

Calcium D-glucarate is a chemical. It is comparable to a naturally occurring chemical called glucaric acid. Glucaric acid is made in our bodies as well as in fruits and vegetables such as oranges, apples, brussels sprouts, broccoli, and cabbage[9].

---

9   C. Dwivedi, W. J. Heck, A. A. Downie, et al, "Effect of calcium Glucarate on B-glucuronidase activity and Glucarate content on certain vegetables and fruits," *Biochemical Medicine and Metabolic Biology* 43 (1990): 83–92.

Calcium D-glucarate is made by combining glucaric acid with calcium to make supplements that people use for medicine in estrogen-related diseases.

It is also used in cancer treatment in estrogen-dependent cancers[10]. It's used for preventing breast, prostate, and colorectal cancer.

To lower estrogens in the body, you should be taking some form of calcium D-glucarate, as this substance essentially mops up the estrogens in the liver's detoxification pathway.

Bodybuilders use this product to ensure lower levels of estrogens and higher levels of testosterone naturally. This helps them burn fat. So why shouldn't overweight people use it? It is a very safe product that helps liver function. We all know what the effects of estrogen reduction are: weight loss and fat burn.

Therapeutic Dose
100–200mg/meal

Test levels of estrogen in the blood and see if the calcium-D-glucarate is effective. Increase the dose accordingly to help lower estrogens further.

Testing Estrogen Levels

As a professional, I would suggest that when you test for estrogens and progesterone, you order a comprehensive hormonal profile (progesterone, estrogens, DHEA, testosterone, etc.) that includes 2 Hydroxyestrone (2OHE) and 16 alpha Hydroxyestrone (16aOHE) and estrogen metabolism ratio. The former is the good "light" estrogen and the latter is the bad "heavy" estrogen.

---

[10] Z. Walaszek, M. Hanausek-Walaszek, J. P. Minton, and T. E. Webb, "Dietary Glucarate as anti-promter of 7,12-dimethylbenz(a)anthracene-induced mammary tumorigenesis," *Carcinogenesis* 7 (1986): 1463–1466.

Bad estrogen such as 16aOHE is a major cause of breast cancer, rheumatoid arthritis, and lupus. Making sure that the basic hormones of the estrogens (E1, E2, E3) and progesterone, as well as testosterone, are balanced as well as keeping the 16aOHE lower in concentration than the 2OHE will keep women free from breast cancer and other autoimmune diseases. This fact also applies to men.

How to Balance Progesterone

Estrogen must be balanced by an opposing hormone called progesterone.

If a woman is prescribed estrogens long-term in the form of birth-control pills or hormone-replacement therapy, or a man, child, or woman eats far too many types of meat laced with estrogen derivatives, the estrogen levels of that individual will start to rise and become out of balance compared to the progesterone. This situation is called **estrogen dominance**. If a man becomes estrogen dominant, then he will get man boobs, a belly, enlarged prostate (BPH), hair loss, and general weight gain with low testosterone.

Ultimately the estrogens and the xenoestrogens set up an imbalance within our system where the progesterone levels become too low, and of course the progesterone-deficiency disease will then manifest (e.g. fibroids, breast cancer, ovarian cancer, endometriosis, prostate problems, hair loss, heart disease, and fertility issues).

Using natural progesterone cream or liquid drops are effective ways to treat men and women who are progesterone deficient. Cream or liquids are the preferred methods of delivery, as this avoids the first pass thorough the liver where it would be prone to breaking down earlier. Creams allow the hormones to stay active for longer.

Therapeutic Dose

You must improve your diet for the progesterone to work, because alcohol, sugar, caffeinated drinks, sweets, cereals, bread, cereal fiber, and milk products all *lower* progesterone activity. Following a blood-type paleo diet, as I wrote about in my first book, *The Hidden Cure*—fruits, vegetables, meat, poultry, eggs, fish, and organic foods—will also improve progesterone levels.

- **Females** = 18–32mg every night for two weeks in the luteal phase of menstruation. Postmenopausal women should cycle three weeks on, one week off. Repeat cycle. Apply one hour before bed on the arms, legs, and chest or breast. For cysts and fibroids, progesterone should be applied vaginally or on the lower stomach. Profemme, bioidentical progesterone cream*/yam-based source. Manufactured by Lawley Pharmaceuticals, Aus.
- **Males** = 5 - 20 mg every night, one hour before bed. Some men need more (>20mg/night) to get rid of their symptoms and occasionally have had to give higher doses initially and then slowly reduce the dose to a maintenance dose of 10mg/night. etc

How to Balance Testosterone

Testosterone opposes the action of estrogen. Anything that raises cortisol stress levels will raise estrogen and lower testosterone.

Testosterone therapy takes time to see results. Most results take about three months to see about 30–40 percent improvements. Monitor to see how the numbers change every three months until you are in the optimal range.

Remember there are strong connections between low testosterone and the development of diabetes, heart disease, and reduced life span. Low-dose testosterone therapy to achieve optimal health and resist disease is not the same as bodybuilding. Bodybuilders take in one month what it would take to treat a low-testosterone male for three to five years. We are looking for optimal health, not an extreme muscular physique.

Natural Therapeutics to Boost Testosterone

Testosterone requires several cofactors in its production, which are listed as follows:

- Vitamin E 400iu
- Lipoic acid 100mg
- Co Q10 30–120mg
- Zinc 50mg
- Vitamin C 1000mg
- L-Arginine 500–1000mg (avoid if there is a history of herpes)
- B complex 50mg
- DHEA 5–15mg (depending on blood/saliva test result and gender)
- Nettle tea (stimulate testosterone production) 1–2 cups per day
- Bioidentical testosterone cream*/yam-based source

Therapeutic Dose:
- Androforte Testosterone Cream for males 5% = 50–100mg/day/three weeks on and one week off. Manufactured by Lawley Pharmaceuticals, Aus.
- Androfemme Testosterone Cream for females 1% = 5–10mg/day/three weeks on and one week off. Manufactured by Lawley Pharmaceuticals, Aus.

Testosterone, fat metabolism and increasing muscle mass[11] are synonymous with each other, and if the level of testosterone can

---

11   Shalender Bhasin, Thomas W. Storer, Nancy Berman, Kevin E. Yarasheski, Brenda Clevenger, Jeffrey Phillips, W. Paul Lee, Thomas J. Bunnell, and Richard Casaburi, "Testosterone Replacement Increases Fat-Free Mass and Muscle Size in Hypogonadal Men," *JCEM* 82 (1997): 407–413.

be returned to optimal range, the results can be quite amazing even in older men[12].

It is a scientific fact that the majority of overweight or obese men have lower testosterone levels, sugar issues, high estrogen, and heart problems compared to slim, fit men. Placing them on a course of low-dose testosterone can safely induce weight loss[13].

Obesity is related to the risk of developing cardiovascular diseases and T2 diabetes. You should test for testosterone to see if it is at its optimal range, i.e. youthful ranges of a man around twenty-five to thirty years of age[14]. I believe that prostate problems and prostate cancer are due to a chronic progesterone and testosterone deficiency. As a caution, men should also test their PSA levels and rule out any prostate cancer on an annual basis.

How to Balance the Thyroid

This section only deals with supplements for thyroid function, and in certain cases your MD may see fit to use a thyroid hormone. Nevertheless, plenty of patients find great success using a natural approach, knowing that they can use the thyroid hormone-replacement therapy as a backup only if absolutely necessary.

---

12 Fred R. Sattler, Carmen Castaneda-Sceppa, Ellen F. Binder, E. Todd Schroeder, Ying Wang, Shalender Bhasin, Miwa Kawakubo, Yolanda Stewart, Kevin E. Yarasheski, Jagadish Ulloor, Patrick Colletti, Ronenn Roubenoff, and Stanley P. Azen, "Testosterone and Growth Hormone Improve Body Composition and Muscle Performance in Older Men," *JCEM* 94 (2009): 1991–2001.

13 W. Faloon, MD, "Physician's guide: Using blood tests to safely induce weight loss," *Life Extension* 15(6) (2009): 42–63.

14 Wald, M., Meacham, R.B., Ross, L.S. et al. "Testosterone replacement therapy for male aging: ASA position statement," *J. Androl.* 27(2) (2006): 133–134.

Treatment for Hypothyroidism

Listed below are some of supplements that we use at our clinic to stimulate the thyroid in our patients:

- Take daily thyroid support with iodine (thyroid complex, armor, tyrosine)
- Kelp, dulse, and seaweed are also good natural sources
- Iodine—1mg/day
- Tyrosine (amino acid)—500-1500mg/day
- Zinc—50-100mg/day
- Vitamin A 500-10,000i.u./day
- Vitamin E 400 i.u./day
- Co Q10 100-300mg/day
- Copper 1-2mg/day
- Selenium 200mcg/day
- B complex 50mg/day
- Thyroid glandular (desiccated)

In some cases the thyroid should be supported with an excellent natural pharmaceutical called Armour Thyroid (Thyrar) Westhroid and Nathroid. These contain desiccated thyroid support from porcine sources. These pharmaceuticals were the standard of thyroid treatment before the synthetic thyroids pharmaceuticals such as Eltroxin (T4) and Synthroid (T4).

Other synthetic drugs contain T3, such as Cytomel and Triostat. Achieving successful and easy weight loss can only come about by choosing the correct thyroid support and carefully monitoring its response with regular feedback from blood tests. Bear in mind that you need optimal ranges to improve your metabolism.

> **KEY POINT:** In any case of a slow thyroid, the adrenals must be supported. If you boost the thyroid alone with no adrenal support, you may experience adrenal exhaustion or failure (insomnia, palpitations, weight loss, diarrhea).

You must understand that the adrenals and thyroid are functionally connected. Your body is like a band, where each organ plays a different instrument to the same music.

Rebuilding the Thyroid with Functional Foods

First, if you have discovered that you have a sluggish thyroid, then I cannot stress enough your need to avoid gluten-based foods such as wheat, oats, barley, rye, millet, etc., and turnips. These are goitregenic foods; in other words, they slow down the metabolic rate of the gland itself by competing against it with certain nutrients. Regularly eating fish from the sea is a good source of iodine and counteracts the development of goiter and most other thyroid disorders.

Cassava, broccoli, cauliflower, brussels sprouts, cabbage, and kale are also goitregenic in large amounts; however, they do have distinct advantage in that they are great boosters to the liver function and the body's detoxification. The advantages far outweigh the disadvantages. They can be used in small amounts.

I tell my patients as long as they are supporting their thyroid adequately with thyroid supplements or medications, then they will continue to get better. Monitoring the thyroid levels would be key.

Second, if you have reduced the above goitregenic foods, make sure you have adequate amounts of thyroid-stimulating foods such as:

- Dulse
- Seaweed salad (Wakame)
- Dark leafy vegetables
- Alaskan salmon
- Herring
- Cod
- Mackerel

- Brazil nuts
- Mustard greens/horseradish
- Iodized sea salt
- Avocado/guacamole (boosts thyroid activity)
- Sardines (check U/A levels: <5-0)

Occasionally some patients may suffer from an autoimmune disorder of the thyroid, and this ought to be managed by a competent endocrinologist and your wellness physician working together for your best interests.

How to Improve Leptin and Adiponectin Levels

Excess insulin (inflammation), leptin, and adiponectin are somehow linked and are important in how we regulate our *appetite and weight*. There are **ten key things** you can do to lose weight by regulating the leptin and adiponectin levels as follows.

1. EXERCISE—Paying close attention to diet and exercise is the solution to lower leptin levels. Studies conducted at Harvard School of Public Health showed that men who exercised the most had lower leptin[15] levels[16]. The men who exercised the least, weighed the most, and ate the most cholesterol-based foods had the highest leptin levels and were tending toward diabetes. As one becomes fatter, the levels of leptin rise, and as regular exercise is performed, the leptin

---

15 A. Shapiro, W. Mu, C. Roncal, K. Y. Cheng, R. J. Johnson, and P. J. Scarpace, "Fructose-induced Leptin resistance exacerbates weight gain in response to subsequent high-fat feeding," *Am. J. Physiol. Regul. Integr. Comp. Physiol.* 295(5) (2008): 1370–1375.[Missing info-full journal name]

16 N. F. Chu, M. J. Stampfer, D. Spiegelman, N. Rifai, G. S. Hotamisligil, and E. B. Rimm, "Dietary and lifestyle factors in relation to plasma Leptin concentrations among normal weight and overweight men," *Int. Journal of Obesity* 25(1) (2001): 106–114.

levels will fall. So in a strange way, exercise is related to appetite; the more one exercises, the better the leptin sensitivity will become.

2. SLEEP WELL—Studies[17] show that when patients sleep well, their levels of insulin[18] and cortisol are better, and this in turn stabilizes the blood glucose, making the brain more sensitive to the levels of leptin coming from fat cells, which in turn allows the balance of adiponectin.

3. AVOID HFCS—Today sugar in our food products has been substituted with high-fructose corn syrup (HFCS), and although sweet, it is a secret ingredient in that it encourages its consumers to eat more by reducing leptin sensitivity[19]. Avoid it completely. Consuming HFCS in beverages plays a major role in the epidemic of obesity[20].

4. READ LABELS—Read the labels of the food you put into your body. HFCS and other artificial sweeteners, preservatives, and colorings can be found in everything from bread and salad dressings to fruit juices and yogurt to make them look tastier. The theory is that sugar always makes food

---

17　Zmrzljak, Ursula Prosenc, and Damjana Rozman. "Circadian regulation of the hepatic endobiotic and xenobitoic detoxification pathways: the time matters." *Chemical research in toxicology* 25, no. 4 (2012): 811-824.

18　Alexandros N. Vgontzas et al, "Sleep apnea and daytime sleepiness and fatigue: relation to visceral obesity, Insulin resistance, and hypercytokinemia," *Journal of Clinical Endocrinology & Metabolism* 85.3 (2000): 1151–1158.

19　Alexandra Shapiro, Wei Mu, Carlos A Roncal, Kit-Yan Cheng, Richard J. Johnson, and Philip J. Scarpace, "Fructose-Induced Leptin Resistance Exacerbates Weight Gain in Response to Subsequent High Fat Feeding," *Am J Physiol Regul Integr Comp Physiol* 295(5) (2008): 1370–1375. [Missing information]

20　George A. Bray, Samara Joy Nielsen, and Barry M. Popkin, "Consumption of high-fructose corn syrup in beverages may play a role in the epidemic of obesity," *The American Journal of Clinical Nutrition* 79.4 (2004): 537–543.

tastier, and, of course, the tastier the food, the more likely customers are to buy the product again. Sugar creates more sales because it creates addiction, an addiction that an internal yeast/bacterial/parasite infection thrives off, which in turn increases the profits for the company producing it.

5. **FISH OILS**—These help to improve glucose handling by the pancreas and heart muscle and therefore indirectly improve leptin and adiponectin levels[21].

6. **AVOID FASTING**—Nothing stresses the body more than fasting, as the body becomes stressed from the *lack* of food. Within thirty-six hours of fasting, levels of leptin will drop by 70 percent or more[22].

7. **EAT REAL FOOD**—Having a diet rich in fish, nuts, and low-GI fruits and vegetables.

8. **DRINK GREEN TEA**—Do this two to three times a day. Green tea fights fat [23]very well (and heart disease and cancer), and in studies it has been shown to increase liver detoxification[24], improve cholesterol levels[25], and fight obesity[26].

---

21 Trevor A. Mori et al, "Effect of fish diets and weight loss on serum Leptin concentration in overweight, treated-hypertensive subjects," *Journal of Hypertension* 22.10 (2004): 1983–1990.

22 Rexford S. Ahima et al, "Distinct physiologic and neuronal responses to decreased leptin and mild hyperleptinemia," *Endocrinology* 140.11 (1999): 4923–4931.

23 Swen Wolfram, Ying Wang, and Frank Thielecke, "Anti-obesity effects of green tea: From bedside to bench," *Molecular Nutrition & Food Research* 50.2 (2006): 176–187.

24 Mousumi Bose et al, "The major green tea polyphenol,(-)-epigallocatechin-3-gallate, inhibits obesity, metabolic syndrome, and fatty liver disease in high-fat–fed mice," *The Journal of Nutrition* 138.9 (2008): 1677–1683.

25 Nurulain T. Zaveri, "Green tea and its polyphenolic catechins: medicinal uses in cancer and noncancer applications," *Life Sciences* 78.18 (2006): 2073–2080.

26 Yung-hsi Kao, Richard A. Hiipakka, and Shutsung Liao, "Modulation of obesity by a green tea catechin," *The American Journal of Clinical Nutrition* 72.5 (2000): 1232–1233.

9. **USE A SUGAR DESTROYER**[27]—*Gymnema Sylvestre* is an ayurvedic herbal medicine used for thousands of years in India to treat hyperglycemia or excess blood sugar. It has also been used to treat sugar cravings by altering the taste sensation of sugar in the tongue receptors. Gymnema does not induce hypoglycemia, i.e. the hypoglycemia reactions that are sometimes seen with the use of insulin or sulfonylurea drugs used to treat diabetes. Gymnema also can be used to treat weight issues and obesity[28]. Gymnema is a very safe herb to take to help control T2 diabetes and aids in the recovery of insulin sensitivity of the body, as it promotes recovery of the pancreas. As a caution, I will advise that taking Gymnema along with insulin might cause your blood sugar to become too low. Monitor your blood sugar closely. The dose of your daily insulin might need to be changed, so inform your MD of your intentions of regaining your blood-sugar control by fixing the pancreas with herbs.

10. **EAT AFRICAN MANGO**—*Irvingia Gabonensis*—scientific analysis of Irvingia extract has shown that it produces a wide range of benefits to improving LR but also helps with diabetes[29,30] as well as atherosclerosis. Irvingia has been shown to help reduce weight by blocking absorption of carbohydrates from the gut and also improves leptin levels by resisting the enzyme that would convert sugar into stored

---

27   Tiwari, Pragya, B. N. Mishra, and Neelam S. Sangwan. "Phytochemical and Pharmacological Properties of Gymnema sylvestre: An Important Medicinal Plant." *BioMed Research International* 2014 (2014).

28   Ibid 27

29   Ngondi JL, Matsinkou R, Oben JE. The use of Irvingia gabonensis extract (IGOB131) in the management of metabolic syndrome in Cameroon. Nutrition J. 2008

30   Ngondi JL, Oben JE, Minka SR. The effect of Irvingia gabonensis seeds on body weight and blood lipids of obese subjects in Cameroon. Lipids Health Dis. 2005 May 25;4:12.

fat. This allows adiponectin to be released from the fat cells, thereby reactivating communication with the brain and allowing the brain/body to reset the fat-burn switch.

Special note about Irvingia Gabonensis

Irvingia has turned out to become the best dietary weight-loss supplement ever found. Compared to other weight-loss supplements, Irvingia holds king. Patients who took Irvingia with or without dieting ended up with impressive weight loss. Those who did diet in combination with the Irvingia lost more weight than those who didn't.

Middle-Age Burnout?

The main function of fat cells, otherwise known as adipocytes, is to store fat calories in the body. The fat contained within the adipocytes are mainly triglycerides. As people age and stress excessively, their tendency to accumulate triglycerides within fat cells increases. The explanation is premature age decline in the adrenal and sex-hormone production, set in a landscape of excess sugar, overeating, and lack of exercise.

Younger people can eat large amounts of calories and can easily burn off the excess and avoid weight gain. However, older people have to watch their caloric intake carefully without putting on the pounds. The explanation for this observation is that the signal network between the adipocytes becomes blunted as we age/stress, and then weight gain happens, especially in the forties, as this is the point when most people's adrenals are burnt out and they feel the effects of Stage 3 and a serious drop in metabolism.

The Ultimate Fat-Cell Commander

There are three command signals from our adipocytes that are crucial in creating a balanced body.

1. Leptin—when released it cuts the appetite[31]
2. Adiponectin—when released it increases insulin sensitivity [32,33]
3. Glycerol-3-phosphate dehydrogenase—when released it converts sugar into triglycerides[34]

As a supplement, Irvingia increases leptin sensitivity, increases adiponectin, and inhibits glycerol-3-phosphate dehydrogenase[35].

As people become *fatter*, leptin resistance *increases*, and ironically fatter people have higher levels of leptin, but it is bonded to a protein associated with inflammation called C-reactive protein (CRP) and therefore *cannot signal* to the brain to switch off the appetite. The leptin and CRP bonded together becomes such a bigger molecule that it can't fit across the blood-brain barrier, thereby preventing the brain from starting the fat burn and instead *signaling* the body to get fatter.

If one reduces the amount of CRP by eating healthy food that is naturally antiinflammatory and combining that with an Irvingia supplement, weight loss can easily be achieved to allow

---

31   J. M. Friedman. "The function of Leptin in nutrition, weight, and physiology," *Nutrition Review* 60(10) (2002): S1–14.

32   B. I. Shand, R. S. Scott, P. A. Elder, and P. M. George, "Plasma Adiponectin in overweight, nondiabetic individuals with or without Insulin resistance," *Diabetes Obes Metab* 5(5) (2003): 349–353.

33   M. Gil-Campos, R. R. Cañete, and A. Gil, "Adiponectin, the missing link in Insulin resistance and obesity," *Clinical Nutrition* 23(5) (2004): 963–974.

34   L. S. Wise and H. Green, "Participation of one isozyme of cytosolic glycerophosphate dehydrogenase in the adipose conversion of 3T3 cells," *Journal Biology & Chemistry* 254 (2) (1979): 273–275.

35   Ibid 153.

the person's brain to recognize the weight issue and react to the leptin, and this in turn allows the release of adiponectin and fat from the fat cells to be burnt as sugar.

Irvingia lowers cholesterol, balances blood sugar, reduces inflammation, and improves heart function and helps the body to burn fat[36]. Doses range from 120–600mg/day.

A warning: Irvingia *significantly* reduces cholesterol and blood-sugar levels; please monitor these changes regularly (daily/weekly).

Diabetics and patients taking statins must work in conjunction with their physician to monitor their progress and recalibrate the drugs or remove them entirely.

So significant are the natural effects of Irvingia[37], I will write this twice...you are going to lose weight, balance your blood sugar, lower your high cholesterol, and overall have less of an appetite easily, and this is directly linked to your stress levels. Keep a good eye on your situation with regular blood-chemistry tests and inform your MD or DO. It will happen[38]. On average patients lose ten to thirteen pounds in five weeks and around twenty-five to thirty pounds in ten weeks[39].

---

36   Judith L. Ngondi, Julius E. Oben, and Samuel R. Minka, "The effect of Irvingia Gabonensis seeds on body weight and blood lipids of obese subjects in Cameroon," *Lipids Health & Disease* 4 (2005): 12.

37   Judith L. Ngondi et al, "IGOB131, a novel seed extract of the West African plant Irvingia Gabonensis, significantly reduces body weight and improves metabolic parameters in overweight humans in a randomized double-blind placebo controlled investigation," *Lipids in Health and Disease* 8.7 (2009)

38   Stephanie Maxine Ross, "African mango (IGOB131): a proprietary seed extract of Irvingia Gabonensis is found to be effective in reducing body weight and improving metabolic parameters in overweight humans," *Holistic Nursing Practice* 25.4 (2011): 215–217.

39   William Faloon, "More Weight Loss than Any Other Discovery in Supplement History," *Life Extension Magazine* (2008). https://www.lef.org/magazine/mag2008/ss2008_report_more-weight-loss.htm

How to Improve Ghrelin Levels

Having meals on time and following a good balanced diet allows the ghrelin levels to rebalance. Keeping some protein in the stomach in between meals is also a good technique. Getting to bed on time (sleeping 10:00 PM–6:00 AM) and having adequate sleep allows the ghrelin to stabilize.

How to Improve Melatonin Levels

This is an easy fix, as it is readily available in tablets and sprays. The more melatonin one takes at night, the deeper the sleep. Once again, balance is key here, and excess levels of melatonin may cause excessive drowsiness, and too little melatonin causes insomnia. Approximately 3mg/night is sufficient. One to three sprits should suffice.

"Let your food be your medicine, and let medicine be your food."

—Hippocrates

Chapter 13

Creating Your Fat-Burning Plate

Paleo-Metabolic Typing

Burning fat is dependent on having two key organs working well, and these are the thyroid and adrenal glands. To "burn fat" well, you need to understand what your metabolism is doing and choose the appropriate food ratios of protein and fats vs. carbohydrates to match your metabolism. Through metabolic typing, you can modify the way your hormones work for the better.

If you don't follow this, then certain fatty foods that you eat could slow you down or speed you up. No guesswork—find out what your metabolic type is, and then you can choose the right food ratios to help nudge your metabolism for the better.

What Is Paleo-Metabolic Typing?

This is a fusion of the paleo diet with the metabolic-type diet that we practice at my clinic. When my patients follow their physiological clues about metabolism and apply the correct proteins for their blood type, excellent improvements in metabolism are noted.

Metabolic typing is a method of evaluating and interpreting your innate pattern of metabolism that determines your individual reaction to foods and nutrients. We all inherit strengths and weaknesses—that is, definite gene patterns of biological and neurological origin—that decide our personal nutritional necessities. This theory is based on the work of William Walcott. If you correct your metabolic imbalance by choosing the right ratios of food, then you will burn fat. Eating only the appropriate blood-type proteins is key.

Paleo-Blood-Type Theory: Scientists have put forward a report that gives a scientific[1] modernized approximation of what diet our "caveman" ancestors may have eaten throughout the time from their initial emergence in Africa some 200,000 years ago. The Paleo-blood-type approach has been compared to the Mediterranean Diet and has shown that it is better at improving metabolism and cardiovascular function overall.

The report shows that our ancestors ate higher percentages of protein, in the region of 25–29 percent, 40 percent carbohydrates, and 30 percent fats. Our paleo ancestors consumed omega oils, according to the report, in relatively moderate amounts of approximately six grams/day in the form of wild game and fish.

What is your blood type tribe? = O - A - B - AB

Putting It into ACTION

Eat only ideal blood-tribe protein[2]. Now that you know what your blood type is you must choose from the ideal protein list.

O Bloods - meat, poultry, fish, eggs, shellfish

A Bloods - poultry, fish, eggs, shellfish

B Bloods - turkey, beef, lamb, fish, eggs

AB Bloods - turkey, fish, lamb, eggs

---

1   Stephanie Jew, Suhad Abu Mweis, and Peter J. H. Jones, "Evolution of the Human Diet: Linking Our Ancestral Diet to Modern Functional Foods as a Means of Chronic Disease Prevention," *Journal of Medicinal Food* 12(5) (2009): 925–934.

2   P. D'Adamo, P (with additional material by Catherine Whitney), Eat Right 4 Your Type (New York: Putnam, 1996),

Eating by Paleo-Metabolic Typing[3]

The ideas and techniques in this section are, primarily, to do with fat metabolism (or fat burn); however, it will also be important for you to work out whether you are a protein or a carbohydrate type (i.e. whether your body needs to eat more carbohydrate foods or protein foods).

If you are a protein type, you will enjoy eating healthy fats with your proteins, and if you are a carbohydrate type, you will enjoy eating healthy fats with your carbohydrates. Sometimes you'll feel like having both (mixed type).

It's important to determine your metabolic type in order to concentrate your diet to encourage greater energy and weight loss. Take the short quiz that follows to reveal your metabolic type tendency.

Metabolic Typing Quiz[4]

Circle your answers to the following questions:

Y or N: Is your appetite at breakfast strong?

Y or N: Is your appetite at lunch strong?

Y or N: Is your appetite at dinner strong?

Y or N: Does eating before bedtime improve your sleep?

Y or N: Do you live to eat and not to subsist?

Y or N: Do you get hungry in between meals?

Y or N: Does fasting make you feel bad?

Y or N: Do you crave salt?

Y or N: Do fatty meals agree with you?

---

3   William Walcott and Trish Fahey, *The Metabolic Typing Diet: Customize Your Diet to Your Own Unique Body Chemistry Crown Publishing Group*, Three Rivers Press, Nov 19, 2008

4   Steve Denk, adapted from the BioMedX training course for Physicians, Chicago, 2001 USA.[missing info]

Y or N: Does skipping meals make you uncomfortable?

Y or N: Does meat or fish at breakfast give you more energy?

Y or N: Does meat or fish at lunch give you more energy?

Y or N: Does meat or fish at dinner give you more energy?

Y or N: Does eating meat or fatty foods restore your energy?

Y or N: Do you feel bloated after meals?

Count up the total of your "yes" answers =

Count up the total of your "no" answers =

Interpretation:

If you have more "yes" answers = protein and fat type diet plate and you lean towards a Parasympathetic type nervous system with slightly lower blood pressure (> 110 / > 70) ~ usually reflects a low energy status and a tendency to feel depressed / low mood

If you have equal "yes" and "no" answers = mixed type diet plate / you have "balanced" nervous system and you lean towards a normal blood pressure (around 120 / 80) ~ balanced mood, balanced energy

If you have more "no" answers = carbohydrate type diet plate / you lean towards a Sympathetic nervous system and you lean towards a higher blood pressure (< 130 / < 90) ~ usually reflects a higher energy status, anxiety, tension, inability to relax

Diagnostic Assessment of Metabolic Type and Meal Suggestions

Follow the suggestions for your category carefully. Please remember your blood-type protein and low-GI-to-moderate-GI carbohydrates. Being able to "juggle" these key areas of carbohydrates, proteins, and fats will allow you to create any metabolism you want or any body type you want.

PROTEIN and FAT PLATE (PARASYMPATHETIC type)

- Approximately 65–70 percent of the meal must be protein and fat, 30–35 percent low-GI carbohydrates.
- You must eat protein and fat with every meal and snack often. This helps to control blood-sugar swings.
- Eat protein sources such as red or dark meats, chicken or turkey with the skin on, nuts, seeds, eggs, and beans.
- You should eat often throughout the day in smaller meals (five times).
- Enjoy eating fats and oils such as butter, coconut oil, and olive oil.
- Eat moderate amounts of vegetables, artichokes, asparagus, avocados, carrots, olives, peas, squash, celery, green beans, and baked beans.
- Avoid high-GI fruits and fruit juices.
- The only fruits allowed are bananas, pears (firm), berries, and apricots.
- You must avoid wheat-, rice-, and sugar-based products.
- Limit your grain consumption.
- Avoid vinegar or remove it completely and use lemon instead.

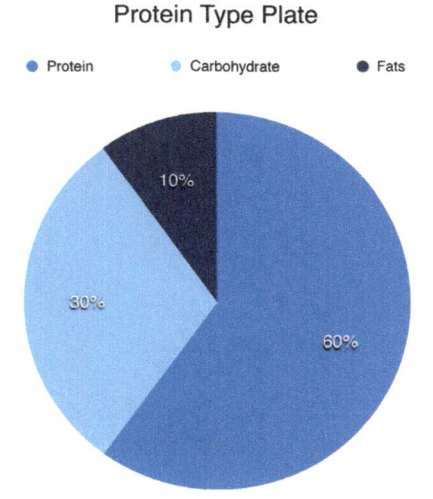

Protein Type Plate

- Protein: 60%
- Carbohydrate: 30%
- Fats: 10%

This is the correct ratio of food for a protein metabolic type.

CARB PLATE (SYMPATHETIC type)

- You should eat approximately 35 percent proteins and fats and 65 percent low-GI carbohydrates at each meal.
- Eat low-fat proteins such as poultry or fish (no red meat).
- Eat plenty of vegetables and salads.
- Enjoy fruits: apples, berries, grapes, pineapple, peaches, and cherries.
- All grains are okay except oats.
- Avoid dairy and butter; they are too high in fat.
- Though you have a high tolerance for sweets and sugary foods, keep high-fat foods to a minimum.
- Carb types have a tendency to rely on caffeine; try to minimize your caffeine intake.
- Eat very few nuts and seeds.

Carbohydrate Type Plate

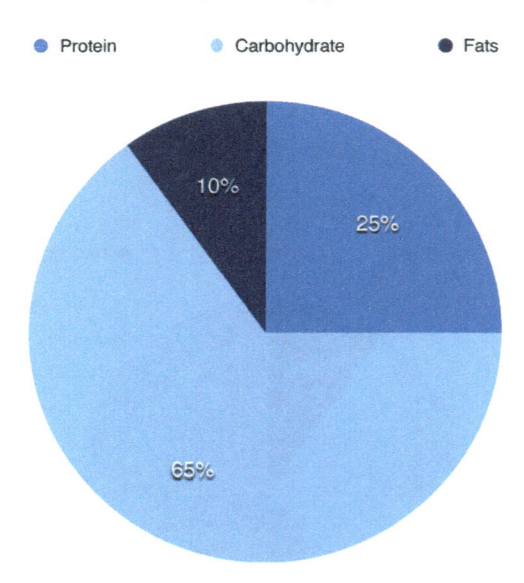

- Protein
- Carbohydrate
- Fats

- 10%
- 25%
- 65%

This is the correct ratio of food for a carbohydrate metabolic type.

MIXED PLATE (BALANCED type)

If you are a mixed type, you require a balance of protein, carbohydrates and fats. You have the broadest menu options of all types.

- Some meals will follow protein-type rules and others will follow the carbohydrate-type rules.
- You are in constant flux—sometimes you will have a huge appetite, yet at other times you will be able to starve for a while.
- Be wary of high-sugar foods, as this will tip you into an acidic pattern that can cause lethargy and yeast development.

If you are a mixed metabolic type, you:

- Should eat 50 percent protein and fat and 50 percent carbohydrates
- Should eat protein at every meal.
- Must eat only blood-type-applicable dairy.
- Should choose low-GI to moderate-GI carbohydrates.
- Must be careful with grains.
- Must avoid bread: eat Ezekiel bread as a better option.
- Should eat fats and oils in moderate amounts.
- Should avoid alcohol, sugar, and caffeine.

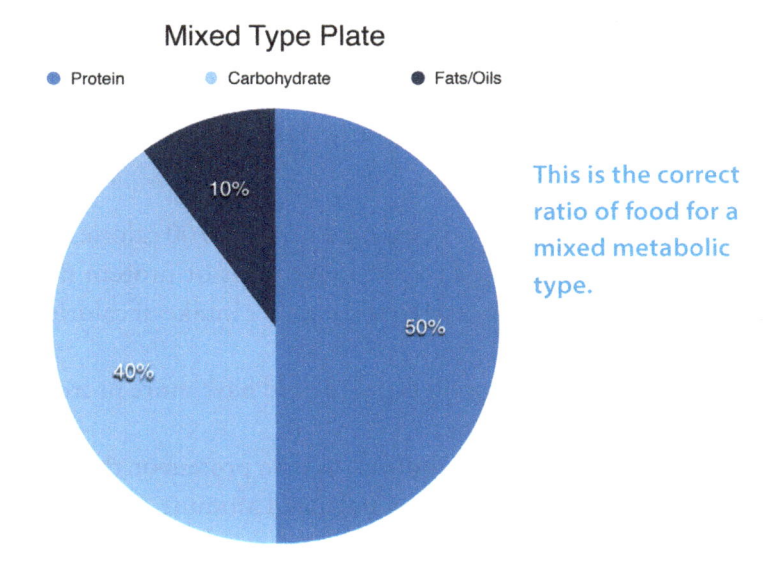

Mixed Type Plate

- Protein
- Carbohydrate
- Fats/Oils

Protein: 50%
Carbohydrate: 40%
Fats/Oils: 10%

This is the correct ratio of food for a mixed metabolic type.

Putting It into Action

Memorize your typical plate ratios. Know what your metabolic type is and plate your food accordingly. The following chart gives you a general idea of how an average day's meal plan should be structured:

MEAL/METABOLIC TYPE	PROTEIN TYPE	MIXED TYPE	CARBOHYDRATE TYPE
BREAKFAST	3 PROTEIN, 1 CARB	2 PROTEIN, 2 CARB	1 PROTEIN, 2 CARB
SNACK (LOW G.I. FRUIT & NUTS)	2 PROTEIN, 1 CARB	2 PROTEIN, 2 CARB	1 PROTEIN, 2 CARB
LUNCH	4 PROTEIN, 1 CARB 2 FATS	4 PROTEIN, 1 CARB 1 FAT	4 PROTEIN, 2 CARB 1 FAT
SNACK (LOW G.I. FRUIT & NUTS)	2 PROTEIN, 1 CARB	2 PROTEIN, 1 CARB	2 PROTEIN, 2 CARB
DINNER	4 PROTEIN, 1 CARB 2 FATS	4 PROTEIN, 2 CARB 2 FATS	4 PROTEIN, 2 CARB 1 FAT

KEY:

1 meal carb = 1 cup of vegetables or ½ cup gluten-free oats

1 snack carb = ½ cup of fruit (low GI)

1 meal protein = 1 oz. of meat, fish or chicken, turkey

1 snack protein = ½ oz. of nuts (raw almonds, Brazil, pecans, sunflower seeds etc.)

1 fat = 1 tbsp of nut butters (almond butter)

1 fat = 1 tsp of olive oil/butter or 1 oz. of avocado or 1 oz. of cheese

N.B The preceding chart is based on a 1,500–1,700 calorie intake, and as such you may need to add more carbs or protein if your calorie calculation shows a need for a higher intake of calories for a carb or protein type.

In other words, a "protein type" should have more protein on their plate than a carb type.

A "carb type" has to have more carbs than protein on their plate.

A "mixed type" has to have a balanced amount.

Now, this is *not* a fixed system. The body can change metabolically and does, and when people become healthy on their metabolic-type diet, they will usually move into a "mixed type" direction. The mixed type is the most balanced out of the groupings and is the natural state of a well-tuned body with a normal blood pressure.

Sugar / HFCS are major Fat Traps

Sugar was once a delicacy that very few people could access or afford. It was used as a treat to flavor cakes and biscuits, and it was added to beer for a fuller flavor. However, sugar is now one of the easiest items to get and appears in most foods bought at the supermarket.

Sugar and high-fructose corn syrup (HFCS) are the secret addictive ingredient in the most unexpected foods[5]. One has to be very aware of the food labels. HFCS can be found in everything from bread and salad dressings to fruit juices and yogurt to make them tastier. The theory is that sugar always makes food tastier, and, of course, the tastier the food, the more likely customers are to buy the product again. Sweet foods create more sales because they create addiction, which in turn increases the profits for the company producing the addictive food. HFCS is clearly linked to leptin resistance and in turn creates hunger and insulin challenges[6]. HFCS makes fat cells larger[7].

The latest statistic from the U.S. Department of Agriculture is that Americans are consuming, on average, in excess of 145 pounds of the stuff every year per person[8].

---

5   Victor Fulgoni, "High-fructose corn syrup: everything you wanted to know, but were afraid to ask," *The American Journal of Clinical Nutrition* 88.6 (2008): 1715S–1715S.

6   Kathleen J. Melanson et al, "Effects of high-fructose corn syrup and sucrose consumption on circulating glucose, insulin, leptin, and ghrelin and on appetite in normal-weight women," *Nutrition* 23.2 (2007): 103–112.

7   Bonnie Jenkins, "High Fructose Corn Syrup-Obesity Sweet Sweet Summer,"

8   Vasanti S. Malik, Matthias B. Schulze, and Frank B. Hu, "Intake of sugar-sweetened

Obesity and diabetes (diabesity) is growing out of control.[9] More kids are being diagnosed with obesity and diabetes than ever before. Kids are now being diagnosed with heart disease and cholesterol problems at earlier ages. The rate of obesity in children has doubled since 1970, and due to this, insurance companies do not want to give medical insurance in some extreme cases. All of this is directly related to the ever-increasing sugar intake beginning at an early age. Now it's time for a natural alternative to sugar—it's called xylose or xylitol.

History of Xylitol/Xylose

Anthropological evidence points toward ancient Siberian shamans who used birch sap for the treatment of many illnesses such as skin diseases, fungal infections, and skin cancer. Living birch trees are resistant to fungal growth when alive, and shamans would harvest the sap as an ointment or syrup/paste to treat skin infections and gut infections.

Medically, xylitol has been proven to be very effective against dental plaque[10,11], prevention of ear infections[12], and treatment of candida infections[13].

---

beverages and weight gain: a systematic review," *The American Journal of Clinical Nutrition* 84.2 (2006): 274–288.

9   Michael I. Goran, Geoff D. C. Ball, and Martha L. Cruz, "Obesity and risk of type 2 diabetes and cardiovascular disease in children and adolescents," *Journal of Clinical Endocrinology & Metabolism* 88.4 (2003): 1417–1427.

10   L. Trahan, "Xylitol: a review of its action on mutans streptococci and dental plaque--its clinical significance," *International Dental Journal* 45.1 Suppl 1 (1995): 77.

11   http://www.drhoffman.com/page.cfm/936

12   Matti Uhari, Tero Kontiokari, and Marjo Niemelä, "A novel use of xylitol sugar in preventing acute otitis media," *Pediatrics* 102.4 (1998): 879–884.

13   Laurens Maas BSc, Ost, DIHom, *The Hidden Cure*- Tucson, Arizona,Wheatmark Press, 2009

Xylitol was discovered in 1891 by a German chemist named Emil Fischer. When sugar was in short supply during World War II due to the effective submarine tactics of destroying cargo ships carrying sugar, the Finns would use xylitol from birch trees.

The consequence was that they had stronger immune systems; lost weight; and had fewer cavities, coughs, colds, and ear infections. Epidemiological studies by the government of Finland confirmed this. As a result of WWII, the world at large benefited from this forgotten secret sugar.

What Is Xylitol, and How Does It Work in the Human Body?

Xylitol is a sugar originally extracted from birch trees. This amazing sugar-replacement molecule is a 5-carbon sugar alcohol otherwise known as a polyol. Glucose is a 6-carbon molecule. Xylitol is a 5-carbon sugar. Its chemical formula is $C_5H_{12}O_5$. It has a glycemic index of 7. Glucose has an index of a whopping 100! Xylitol is synthesized from birch trees, fibrous fruits, vegetables, and corncobs.

The chemical formula is identical to the natural formula, and as such the compound is regarded by the World Health Organization and the FDA as generally safe for human consumption.

N.B It is a very stable compound, but even small amounts of xylitol can be toxic to dogs, so if you add it to your food, **do not** give your scraps to your pets.

Xylitol is a white crystalline powder. That in itself makes it appear synthetic; however, it is completely natural. It's white because the sap of the birch trees or corn syrup is very similar to maple syrup, which also has a glassy consistency.

Xylitol has 40 percent fewer calories compared to ordinary sugar, but it has the same level of sweetness. It is metabolized as a carbohydrate, but it does not require insulin for its management. The human body actually produces between ten and fifteen grams per day of xylose sugar for its daily metabolism. Yes, xylose is actually made by the human body.

Xylitol and Humans

Xylitol is great as a sweetener. It is metabolized into glycogen, the stored form of sugar/glucose in the liver and in the muscles. It's good for bodybuilders in that it is anabolic to the muscles and catabolic to fat. It requires no insulin function and therefore cannot start an anabolic reaction of fat gain.

Bacteria and fungi such as streptococcus and candida cannot metabolize xylitol because of its 5-carbon structure. It's a powerful antimicrobial. It can also be used as an irrigator to treat sinus infections and helps prevent ear infections in children. Plenty of studies have shown that regular use with xylitol prevents dental caries and reduces bad breath.

Xylitol increases the efficiency of the gut by inhibiting yeast in the guts, and therefore the amount of vitamins and minerals absorbed increases.

Disadvantages of Xylitol

When introducing xylitol into the diet, there is a time of adaptation by the gut. If too much is consumed per day, the temporary side effects include loose stools and gas. However, plenty of my patients who suffer from constipation enjoy it for those properties.

While unknown in many overseas countries, primarily because cheap supplies of sugar cane dominate the market, xylitol is slightly more expensive than cane sugar. However, in light of recent evidence that clearly shows the harmful effects of sugar, the general public may feel that the extra money spent on xylitol will keep them in better health. Good health saves money in the long run.

N.B: Alternative to xylitol/xylose is another natural sweetener called erythritol, which does not cause any loose stools.

Advantages of Xylitol Over Other Sweeteners

The clear advantages of xylitol have been shown. It leaves the artificial sweeteners in its dust. No other sweetener has so many benefits to its consumers. Xylitol is completely natural; humans actually manufacture it inside their bodies already.

- Xylitol is antimicrobial and it stops and kills candida and bacteria.
- Xylitol encourages weight loss by stabilizing insulin.
- Xylitol balances sugar levels and is good for hypoglycemic patients.
- Xylitol is safe for diabetics because it requires no insulin.
- Splenda has been proven to carry a chlorine molecule that pickles the nervous system, which over time can sedate the nervous system and pancreas (chloroform, an anesthetic, is used for it's sedative qualities).
- Aspartame turns into formaldehyde, which will pickle the liver.
- Saccharin tastes bad and very artificial.
- Even stevia has an aftertaste and also has no valid energy release.

With all its fantastic properties, xylitol can compete strongly in today's market due to the fact that there is a clear trend of consumerism that shows more and more people will spend their dollars and cents on good, healthy foods that prevent disease. Xylitol is one such natural sugar; it's a functional food.

Summary

- Eat yeast- and gluten-free low-GI foods (xylitol).
- Eat correct paleo-blood-type-diet proteins.
- Eat by metabolic type—carb vs. protein ratio.
- Eat your veggies and supplement your minerals.
- Support your adrenals with supplements, glandular and yam extracts.
- Support your deficient sex hormones with natural bioidentical hormones—progesterone and testosterone.
- Support your thyroid with supplements, glandular and iodine.
- Take a daily amount of Irvingia/African mango extract.
- Take a daily amount of Gymnema Sylvestre.
- Take a nightly amount of melatonin if necessary.

Next we will learn how to exercise and how to think to achieve our goals. Once the stress is lower and the hunger is under control, we can then apply a solid, scientifically proven approach to building muscle with exercise and natural hormone optimization.

CHAPTER 14

Strong Body

Warning—*Before embarking on any exercise program, you should have an evaluation performed by a competent physician (MD, DO, DC, ND) to check your fitness level. This creates a good opportunity to get some blood tests, hormone panels, and an idea of how intense your early fitness sessions can be.*

Ever admired an athlete's great physique? I have. Fit and healthy bodies are very desirable because the life force is boosted. Athletes have great physiques due to the fact that they have hormones that are already in great balance. If you want a good body and energy levels, then getting great hormone levels is a good start.

Athletes also have great physiques because of their sporting lifestyle and *meticulous* diet. We can all learn from their lifestyles, and fortunately for us, we don't have to spend as many hours in hard physical training! While their careers depend on an impeccable physique, most of us would be happy with just looking our best. We can use some of their trade secrets regularly to develop a good body with a lower percentage of body fat and lots of energy.

Before getting to the levels of elite training of an athlete, remember athletes have the same normal-functioning pancreas, adrenals, and thyroids as your potential recovery. If you're following this program, it is very important to get those glands moving into optimal ranges with the help of the supplements suggested or the professional advice of your holistic physician.

When the athlete gets familiar with the same exercise routine and no more muscles are grown, this is called an exercise plateau. Good trainers and coaches will mix up the training routines regularly every three to four weeks to help break up the plateau effect. Doing this creates a state of "muscle confusion."

This concept has been thoroughly explored by celebrity trainer Tony Horton of the USA. Exercise plateaus are when the body gets used to or familiar with a certain level of training. By changing the duration, intensity, and type of exercise, the muscles of the body have to be rebuilt, which in turn causes the body to produce more growth hormone and testosterone, which is essential to building muscle and burning fat.

Some athletes even stop training for a week to give the body a complete rest, as overtraining can cause adrenal disorders[1] and the dreaded burnout. Overtraining can lead to adrenal burnout[2]. I advise my athletes to get soft-tissue massages regularly, as that maintains flexibility and strength, and to be careful to avoid overtraining. Each athlete I have had the fortune to treat for adrenal burnout—from eleven-time world surfing champion Kelly Slater back in 2005 to Olympian swimmers and track-and-field stars to world-class cricketers and tennis champions—has regularly done one or more of the following to help with their overall physique:

Pilates—The ability to have a strong core is key to the development of balanced muscles. Controlled muscular balance between all muscle groups creates fantastic tone.

Yoga or Stretching—The ability of have muscles that are strong depends on them being flexible.

Bodybuilding—Exercises to the large muscle groups create energy and powerful workouts that in turn build metabolic energy. Key areas that are concentrated with interval training are as follows:

---

[1] M. J. Lehmann et al, "Training and overtraining: an overview and experimental results in endurance sports," *Journal of Sports Medicine and Physical Fitness* 37.1 (1997): 7–17.

[2] Jeremy Adams and Robert Kirkby, "Exercise dependence and overtraining: The physiological and psychological consequences of excessive exercise," *Sports Medicine, Training and Rehabilitation* 10.3 (2001): 199–222.

- Leg workouts—squats, lunges, and knee extensions
- Chest and Shoulder workouts. Upper-body strength in the arms comes from having strong shoulders. Shoulder exercises automatically involve both triceps, biceps, and chest muscles

Swimming—This is a complete workout, as it involves all muscle groups while being very low-weight-bearing on all the joints.

Tabata—This is an exercise protocol for "really fit" athletes from Japan. Designed by an exercise physiologist, it is one of the fastest ways of getting really fit and shredded. This is a protocol designed for athletes. It is a super-aerobic workout:

- Only takes eight to ten minutes every three days, and it turns the body into a fat-burning machine. It is composed of five-minutes of warm-ups, eight minutes of twenty-second maximum-muscle-intensity exercises, followed by ten seconds of rest with a two-minute cooldown. Tabata helps to burn off glucose in the blood rapidly, and then the body has to burn fat.
- CAUTION when approaching Tabata: Use a heart-rate monitor to track the heart rate, as Tabata causes your heartbeats per minute to skyrocket to more than two hundred BPMs. Work with a personal trainer, as this is serious exercise.

Before embarking on an exercise program, please confirm with your holistic physician or wellness MD that your body is ready for exercise and that your thyroid and adrenals are getting in better shape. A simple physical examination and a cardiovascular assessment will confirm this. Exercise can be a real lifestyle change, so it's wise to make sure that your body is ready.

Choose the workout that you will enjoy the most, and add one of the athletic secrets to it. For instance, run on a treadmill followed by yoga or swimming the next day, or go to the pilates studio followed by yoga the next day. Creating variety both in the type of workout and its duration will set up more muscle confusion and thereby create further muscular change. Work the body; use the muscles, alternate building them and resting them; eat sensibly; and sleep well, and you'll make an improvement in your fitness.

Athletic Fat-Burning Secrets

Lift Weights to Lose Weight

The most surprising thing that I have realized over the years of training that I have done in the gym (more than twenty-four years) is the idea that people need to really push the workout routines *for hours* to lose weight. This is simply not true. From all my osteopathic studies, research, and experience, I have learned that to lose weight and burn fat, one needs to exercise regularly two or three times a week. I have also learned that whole body movements using strength-training techniques encourage greater muscularity, weight loss, and fat burn.

The Total Fat Cure is based on the idea that in order to lose fat fast, one needs to increase the metabolic rate of the body and its muscles, and this depends on your adrenal and thyroid hormones. Muscles themselves are the *most* metabolically active tissue other than the human brain and heart. Muscles depend on you to make intelligent food choices and ensure optimal hormone function, especially testosterone. You can only build muscle with a certain amount of testosterone.

In opposition to testosterone, the global environment has been over-estrogenized by pharmaceuticals and mass farming through the mechanism of obesogens. As everybody absorbs more estrogens from their food and pharmaceuticals (birth control/growth promoters), the rest of the world gets sicker, fatter, more cancerous, and diabetic. Nudging up testosterone levels to optimal ranges is an important antidote, as it helps to burn fat and build muscle. However, muscles also need an outside stimulus to grow: exercise. So what is the best technique to make muscles grow fast and burn fat? Muscle-failure techniques are the fastest process to build muscle quickly while the workout duration is usually never more than thirty minutes per workout.

Muscle Failure Creates a Better Fat Burn

By increasing the size of the muscles and limiting carbs to low- and moderate-GI foods, the muscles have no choice but to burn fat. The basic exercise routine best for achieving maximum muscle growth is to perform a set of exercises that causes the muscle to grow. These are exercises that induce temporary muscle failure by the eighth, ninth, or even tenth repetition. It doesn't matter really at which rep the muscle failure is induced, so long as there is a sense of "I can't do one more rep, my muscles are exhausted." The key tactic is to make sure the appropriate weight or resistance band has been chosen. The best way to create strength in the muscles is to do fewer reps somewhere in the region of six to ten reps.

Do fewer repetitions for bigger muscles. Be comfortable and tune in to your muscles and feel the pump, squeeze the muscles, get vascular.

My personal favorite amount of reps is actually eight reps twice a week per body part (biceps, triceps, chest, back, legs), and then the next week it will be ten reps. This allows me to create small amounts of muscle confusion, even on a weekly basis.

Muscle failure, which is a sign that the muscle has been totally exhausted of its glucose supply, will cause the muscle to grow stronger. By reducing the glucose supply in the blood, the muscle has to start breaking down the fat molecules as a means of energy. Lifting heavier weights with low reps is the best way to achieve this. The lower the reps and the heavier the weight is, the more myofibrils develop and the stronger you will become.

As you get fitter, then add more sets, such as an extra set per month to a maximum of three sets. The first month of training is one set per muscle group, the second month is two sets per muscle group, and of course the third month is three sets per muscle group.

Within ninety days there will be a substantial difference in the shape of your body and overall muscularity and fitness.

Free Weights

The traditional approach to strength training is to use free weights. Dumbbells and barbells are the usual choice and have been time-tested by bodybuilders. They allow the body to increase the size of the muscles and therefore burn fat.

Choosing the correct weight is key to inducing temporary muscle failure. For example, if I choose a weight for a set of dumbbell curls, I will use a weight that I can easily curl to about the seventh rep, and then the eighth rep becomes harder, the ninth is even harder, and the tenth is so difficult that I almost cannot complete the set. But I can just about do it, and that's the limit. If you can't do the set, make sure you have a spotter or training partner who will assist you to get through the set.

Resistance Bands

Resistance bands are a great way to work out, especially if you travel and have no time to visit an unfamiliar gym. They are so convenient that they can be used at home or even in a hotel room. When working out with bands, bear in mind that unlike free weights, the tension in the bands is constant, which makes it feel as if you have to create more effort.

With free weights, you know how much you're lifting, but with bands you have to tune in and feel the tension. Choosing the right tension for your workout is key. With resistance bands, you can create more variety in the exercise movements, thereby creating more muscle confusion and better muscle growth.

For example, I will use the highest-resistance band and test to see if I can make six, seven, eight, nine, or ten repetitions and no more. If this is easily achieved, I will either shorten the distance of the band movement by taking up more slack using my feet or use a stronger resistance band, or even try two or three resistance bands at the same time, like when I do my squats or shoulder military press.

To increase the resistance with one band, I will step wide with my feet onto the resistance band and shorten the "slack" even more by spreading my legs apart. Finding the right distance takes practice, but once you have an idea of what's right for you and the level of resistance you want, please memorize that distance or order a higher-resistance band when you get stronger. I bought a kit of five different bands, all color-coded for different levels of resistance.

This type of training causes the muscle fibers to tear and rebuild over the succeeding twenty-four to forty-eight hours (depending on age and hormones). After the repair process has taken place, the muscles are a little stronger.

That said, you must then adjust the weight/resistance band so that it is slightly more difficult the next time you do the exercise. You want to confuse your muscles by causing the body to produce more testosterone and growth hormone.

With this principle of increasing the weights as the muscle heals, the body's metabolic rate starts to increase. If you keep your caloric intake the same and the exercise is slowly ramped up over the weeks, you will have no choice but to burn fat. Ultimately the "ramp up, burn fat" principle must be adapted to all the major muscle groups during the process of training.

Technique is everything, so methodical, slow movements with full concentration are required to get the maximum benefit. So take at least three, four, or even five seconds for each maneuver.

Slow and graceful up until the end of the set, until you start to growl and grunt and sweat starts to pour down your face.

Avoid injuries at all costs by *choosing* the right weight or resistance band and resting in between sessions. If done properly, the muscles will grow and the flab will melt away.

An Ideal Fat-Burning Gym Workout

The ideal workout should be around thirty to forty minutes, including your foundational warm-up session on a treadmill. Make sure you drink pure water during the workout. Rest sessions between the sets should be around ten to twenty seconds (not longer). Just do it and feel the difference.

Remember to ramp up your weights as necessary in order to continue the muscle metabolism and muscle confusion. Here are some suggestions that work well to create muscle confusion:

- Change the order of the workout, e.g. legs, back, biceps etc.
- Increase the duration of the workout, e.g. twenty to forty minutes.
- Change the intensity of the workout, e.g. ramping up the weight of the dumbbells/machines or increasing the resistance bands.
- Change the frequency of the workout, e.g. two or three or four times per week as fitness increases.

Most important: Get a full body massages weekly, as this will loosen the muscle fibers and thereby increases strength. Real athletes get massages regularly.

The quick and ideal workout would be as follows:

Warm-up to get the blood moving

- Bicycle ten to fifteen minutes; mix up the speeds and create variety.
- Or treadmill ten to fifteen minutes, with walking/running intervals between 4 and 6 mph.

- Or NordicTrack ten to fifteen minutes; mix up the speeds and create variety.

Muscle Building—Less Is More

- Biceps curl (wrist rotations)
  1–2 sets of 6–10 reps
- Triceps extension
  1–2 sets of 6–10 reps
- Shoulder/military press
  1–2 sets of 6–10 reps
- Chest bench press/push-ups
  1–3 sets of 6–10 reps
- Back/lat pull-downs or seated rowing
  1–3 sets of 6–10 reps
- Leg squats
  1–2 sets of 6–10 reps
- Leg lunges
  1–2 sets of 8–10 reps
- Calf raises
  1–2 sets of 8–10 reps

Abdominals: Options for Developing Your Core!

- Three sets of ten very careful sit-ups, flexed at the hip (must be done slowly_
- Three sets of twenty to fifty knee raises (standing, alternate between lifting knees to waist level)
- Use isometric abdominal contractions when you can. Just contract your abs while you're waiting in line for the bus or train queue so that you maintain tone periodically through the day.
- Do pilates 100s (only if you have a healthy back). These charge up and tone the abdominals quite quickly.
- Swimming in backstroke also tones up the abdominal muscles. Swim ten to fifteen minutes of backstroke weekly, as this helps to tighten your core.

- Contour abdominal belt—electro-muscle stimulation (EMS or eStim)—devices generate electrical impulses that trigger an action potential in muscle nerve fibers (motor neurons). This is done by sending small, safe electrical impulses to the abdominal muscles via specially designed, medical-grade electrodes that stick onto the surface of the skin. If the abdominal muscles are weak, the amount of stimulated contraction can be easily controlled.

Water: The Life-Giving Liquid

Water is the primary ingredient in all fitness and weight-loss programs. Just having a dry mouth doesn't tell us when we are thirsty. By the time we have a dry mouth, the damage of dehydration has already been done. On a cellular level, water creates all the electricity needed for energy, and without it we would die. Water nourishes our bodies on all levels, from the neurotransmitters in our brain to the detoxification of our livers and kidneys. It cools us down when we are hot, it lines our lungs and helps us breathe, and it is the essential component of blood (80–82 percent), saliva ,and urine.

Research has shown that as we age, our ability to recognize that we are thirsty slowly diminishes, and that of course can lead to chronic stress response and create premature degenerative diseases. Chronic dehydration is pandemic in the world today, and so many diseases can be influenced for the better by drinking enough water. Dehydration causes our bodies to:

- Build up toxins within the organs and tissues
- Have low oxygen transfer between the cells (hypoxia)
- Shut down the immune system
- Reduces muscle strength as muscles are composed largely of water
- Worsen the signs of arthritis

Athletes are well aware of the importance of water because rehydration causes us to become stronger. One 6–8 oz. glass every hour is an excellent guideline. Drinking more water is an absolute necessity when training to cool the body and rehydrate the cells. Some of my athlete patients drink up to three to four liters per day!

Athletes also avoid caffeinated beverages due to the dehydration effect they create. They also spend extra money on making sure that they drink the purest water available. They use filters on their faucets and always carry water with them on training sessions. Athletes rehydrate after training hard because they know that the muscles will reinflate stronger by using amino acids and water. Without water, the muscles cannot repair and fat cannot be burnt because the liver uses water to flush out the waste products of fat metabolism.

Alcohol Is the Urine of Yeast!

Only three creatures have the DNA to make alcohol, and these are yeast, fungi, and cancer cells. Alcohol, I tell my patients, is the urine of yeast. This usually gets them to start thinking better about avoiding it if they want to get fit and lean. Alcohol stops the fat-burning process because it is a refined simple carb.

The human body can only burn fat or burn carbs. It cannot do both. Athletes in serious training will avoid alcohol without exception, as it is detrimental to fat burning, performance, and fitness.

Drink Like an Athlete

There are two key rules that athletes use:
1. Drink plenty of water—before, *during*, and after training.
2. Drink no alcohol (unless celebrating a victory, and even then only two to three units per session).

Eat Like an Athlete

Starving the body will slow down the metabolism. As already mentioned, research shows that the thyroid T3 will decrease when the body detects a starvation process and leptin levels start to lower. The point is that you must eat the correct low- to moderate-GI foods, the correct amount of proteins and vegetables, and keep your hormones in tip-top shape.

When any athlete comes to see me, I always ask what they eat and how they eat. Frequently most will eat the correct way to create a lean, muscular body—five to six smaller meals per day. This is exactly how they create energy. By doing this, the athlete will create a metabolic furnace that will cause the body to shed fat and build muscle.

> **KEY POINT:** Ridiculous as this may sound, eating smaller meals more frequently will increase your body's metabolism. You'll have to try it to believe it as you see the results.

By pushing smaller meals more frequently into the body, the body will respond by having more energy (however, this is only possible if the patient has a stable insulin level, normal thyroid function, and optimal adrenal and sex hormones).

By eating frequently, the athlete will be able to evaporate the molecules of their food and drive the chemical reactions that are needed to build muscle.

By eating *frequently every three hours,* the insulin levels will be maintained and the sugar roller coaster prevented. The highs and lows of insulin are detrimental to weight loss because the body encourages fat-cell deposition.

22 Top Foods for Athletes (Depends on Paleo laws)

1. Eggs—builds muscle tissues fast and is the purest form of protein

2. Salmon, Mackerel, or Herring—loads of omega oils
3. Beef—contains CLA that helps to shed fat
4. Turkey—contains tryptophan that improves mood and sleep
5. Chicken—contains arginine and ornithine that help growth and recovery
6. Natural Yogurt—keeps the colon healthy
7. Broccoli and Other Cruciferous Vegetables-improves liver function
8. Olive Oil—cleans the arteries, great for the skin
9. Garlic—fights fungus and bacteria
10. Berries—powerful antioxidants that protect against aging
11. Flax Seeds—keep testosterone higher, great for arteries and heart
12. Turmeric and Cumin—powerful anti-inflammatory
13. Bananas or Coconut Water—contain potassium that lowers blood pressure and relaxes muscles post-workout
14. Cayenne Pepper—boosts kidney function
15. Chewing Gum—between meals prevents snacking and keeps the digestive enzymes working (do not chew gum if you have a history of stomach ulcers)
16. Grapefruit—between meals this binds and emulsifies fat
17. Green Apples—between meals these bind fat and are low-GI
18. Pine Nuts—these contain an appetite-suppressing ingredient
19. Flax Seed or Linseed Oils—increase satiety and stabilize testosterone
20. Salads Full of Crunchy Fiber—fill the stomach up quickly
21. Vegetable Soup—liquid weighs more than food and contains fewer calories

22. Pure Water—drink pure water as only *pure* water is necessary for weight loss to flush out the *toxins* effectively within the fat cells

23. Being Hungry for an Hour Before Your Next Meal—Sometimes it just means that the body is signaling that it's taking calories from burning fat. Drink some water and wait until food is served. However, eat on schedule, be regular, no delays.

Chapter 15

Strong Mind

Eat Slowly to Shrink the Stomach

"Fast food" is a highly popular craze, but it can mean more than "meals made quick." Eating fast can also mean unnecessary weight gain. Your belly needs to communicate to your brain when it's full so that your brain can stop you from overeating. Taking your time to finish a meal gives enough time for the message to reach the human brain and for an appropriate level of satiety or satisfaction to be communicated.

Even if you're eating at a restaurant, you should eat slowly, setting the course of the meal over forty-five minutes or so. If you're going to have an appetizer and a main course, appreciate the time you have before your entrée arrives. The appetizer will leave you feeling more full if you give yourself time to digest it. Having a small appetizer before the main meal (at least twenty to thirty minutes) will start the satiety hormone signal, and it can help you to eat less at the main course.

❱ **KEY POINT: Eat slowly and wait at least twenty minutes before eating any more food. This gives enough time for the brain to register the food that is actually in the stomach.**

Pace yourself, and you'll be less likely to gain weight. Pausing and patience will allow you to avoid overfilling the stomach. If you eat too much, you will stretch your stomach walls and its stretch receptors, which will in turn demand greater and greater amounts of food to fill it. Food pushes on the sides of stomach, and the brain signals satisfaction with the amount eaten as it gets stretched.

Basically, if the stomach bag is overly stretched and loses its elasticity, more food is needed to activate the "I'm full" feeling. When you drink lots of bubbly soft drinks and beer, which are heavy liquids, stomach laxity really goes out of control. The gases push the stomach like a balloon, warping the stomach receptors. Combine this with a yeast infection, and you could become a voracious eater, stacking on the carbohydrates that then turn into alcohol and fat.

Sure, we want to shed fat and drop a pant size or two, but sometimes we also need to shrink what's on the inside: our stomach. Shrinking your stomach walls will allow you to retune your belly-to-brain receptors to limit you to a smaller volume of food.

I suppose to some degree this would explain the popularity of Lap-Band surgeries amongst obese patients, because it forces them to eat less. A Lap-Band surrogates the missing "I'm full" signals from the stomach-wall receptors.

Mind Over Matter Is the Answer

> **KEY POINT:** Many diet books don't take the emotional and psychological aspect of weight loss into consideration, but the mind is a powerful player in determining the success or downfall of your program.

In traditional Chinese medicine (TCM), the pancreas gland is the seat of two key emotions, namely self-esteem and self-control. This gland is key in the recovery of weight issues and diabetes. According to TCM theory, by getting stability in this gland, one's self-esteem and self-control will get better and better. Matter over mind.

Most patients understand that being overweight makes you unhappy and unhealthy. In life we think first and then we act. The law of cause and effect plays a role here. If we think negatively on a cause level, then we will create the negative effect, e.g. weight gain, diabetes. Mind over matter.

Most diabetic, obese, and overweight patients have issues with self-control and self-esteem. The irony is that when they lose their self-esteem, they lose their self-control and then eat the wrong foods for comfort, often favoring higher-GI foods to get the serotonin rush (happy hormone effect), which in turn (because there are usually higher-GI foods) will also cause further weight gain. As you heal your adrenal glands, the self-esteem will rise as the body's energy rises.

Creating the Right State of Mind for Success

This book is going to describe some of the reasons for weight gain and diabetic issues that go way beyond the ordinary nutritional reasons. There are hormonal influences (which we will cover shortly), but there are also mental reasons for weight gain and diabetes. To achieve success in this program takes more than just following instructions about diet changes and vitamins. This lifestyle change allows you to take full responsibility for how you think and to regain your self-control!

The mental aspect is one of the most important processes to this program because your body won't think "thin" if your mind hasn't decided to do it in the first place. Action follows thought.

Creating vivid images and feelings of how healthy and fit you want to be will carry you into that future. Your thoughts become your reality.

This is one of the key aspects determining the success of the program. The ability to change your mind and make it more powerful so that success is achieved physically is paramount. If you skip this step, then mentally you will not be prepared for success, so set yourself serious mental goals.

The Law of Attraction

Your thoughts are a magnet, attracting the things that you think and feel. This also includes your subconscious thoughts. All energy is constantly in a state of change. It takes energy to change your body shape. It takes energy to change your pancreas. It takes energy to change anything. Interestingly enough, we humans know how to manipulate energy so that we can create a certain outcome. By changing your thinking about food, you will create new tasty dishes for yourself that will improve your body shape and improve your sugar-handling ability.

Your thoughts about food have a particular effect. If you have been struggling with your weight and your diabetic control, then this is an effect of your thinking. Just as the law of cause and effect is a universal law, so is the law of attraction.

You can use the law of attraction to get a better and healthier body by really thinking and meditating about the desired goal. Looking at images of fitter and slimmer people with well-toned bodies will spark your desire to get one of those bodies. By thinking deeply with a passion and emotion, your subconscious mind will start to pay attention to your desires and in turn will help you to fulfill those desires. By being consistent in your meditations and contemplations, your wish can become true. The law of attraction was thoroughly explored through the hit movie *The Secret*.

In the movie the universe's most powerful law was revealed to audiences around the world, showing how the law of attraction can create positive change in people's lives. As the movie says, the power of love and gratitude will dissolve all negativity.

Love can cure any disease, and love is always found within the balance of the mind and the body. Get into the feeling of loving your new body. Be passionate about exercise and training, because it will make you feel and look good.

Avoiding Negative People

Experience has led me to discover that this is an important area of concern. Negative people will foster depression in situations and often feel justified in giving their reasons for a lack of motivation. Negative people will view your new health program with disdain and try to damage your success by giving negative comments with remarks such as, "Oh, go on just have one, it won't hurt you" or "Vitamins just make expensive urine" or the worst one, "How can you give up all those delicious foods without feeling you're missing out?" These kinds of people are being unsupportive, and you must minimize encounters with them.

Focus on being with people who are supportive of your will to get healthy. Positive people around you will foster a state of mind conducive to greater success.

Eliminate Negative Thinking!

Most people have repeatedly negative thoughts. My patients tell me they consistently tell themselves they are fat and they hate the way the look. They are obsessed with it and repeat the same thought processes again and again on a daily basis.

Flip this negative pattern around. You will achieve the results you want by using *positive self-dialogue*. I ask my patients to catch themselves when they talk negatively to themselves and to say something much more positive, such as, "I am getting healthier and I am feeling good on this program, and I am becoming slimmer with each meal and workout." Positive self-dialogue is a must.

Be Specific About Your Goals

Most patients who come to see me for weight loss know what they want, and yet when I ask them what they would look like, there is very little detail.

I explore this area with them so that we both know exactly how the patient will look and feel when they have achieved their goal. I want them to go through the details for their subconscious benefit. Then I get them to write down five key things that they want from themselves through my program. I tell them to be specific and to go into detail. To achieve this I use Neuro-Linguistic Programming (NLP).

Neuro-Linguistic Programming—NLP

One of the best things that I did in my life was to learn how to communicate well, and of course I learned from some of the best communicators in the business, Dr. Richard Bandler and John La Valle. These guys hold fantastic courses in the art of communication, and if you're serious about setting goals and getting what you want out of life, I would suggest doing one of their fabulous courses.

In life, the more effective the communication is, the better the outcome. That means getting what you want depends on how you communicate to yourself and others. The ability to do anything requires a form of communication from our brains to our muscles. More complex human relationships require language, and miscommunication accounts for a lot of failures. And the reverse is also true, in that good communication creates great relationships.

Moving the Donkey—Sticks and Carrots

All permanent change takes place on a psychological level first, and when you have made up your mind, your body and heart will follow. Emphasize the positive and exaggerate it. Use the pain or sticks to drive you forward in your fat-burn program, always knowing what you will achieve as you become slimmer. Use the pain to fuel your desire for change. Imagine regularly how you want your body shape and overall health to look like. Practice this daily, because with practice comes success.

The Stick = Pain

- The psychological pain of being overweight
- The psychological pain of being "socially invisible," low self-esteem
- The psychological pain of being unattractive
- The physical pain of the extra weight on the lower back, hips, and knees
- The organic pain of higher blood pressure, heart problems
- The risk of diabetes
- The economic medical costs of being continuously unhealthy
- The painfulness of exercise (overexercising is stressful to the body and causes a block to the fat-melting process)

The Carrot = Pleasure

- The psychological joy of being slim
- The psychological joy of good self-esteem
- The psychological joy of being more attractive to people
- The physical joy of being fit, with minimal physical pain
- The mental and physical confidence of having a good body
- Much lower medical costs
- The pleasure of exercise, the post-training "high" that comes from it (overexercise is to be avoided)

I advise my patients to exercise *regularly and moderately* two to three times per week. When exercising, mull over the ideas of why you are doing it. Putting mental energy into what you want physically helps to get your subconscious mind aligned with your conscious mind. Meditate on becoming healthier with a slimmer, trimmer body.

An Easy NLP Exercise

What follow are a few key questions that you need to ask yourself before you start this nutritional lifestyle program. Write your answers down in the area allocated. This will prime up your subconscious mind to what you desire. Create pictures of how you *want* to look. Action follows thought.

Here are some questions to get you thinking about your antidiabetic and/or weight-loss goals.

Is your goal stated in positives?

Negative statements do not work well with the subconscious mind, because everything *is possible* in the subconscious mind, because it is holistic and intuitive.

The label of *weight loss* to some people conjures up a sense of loss, which in turn creates a negative response, whereas becoming *slimmer and trimmer* creates a positive response. Transformation is both mental and physical. Write down what your health goals are in a positive way here.

Answer: _____
_____
_____
_____
_____
_____
_____
_____
_____
_____
_____
_____
_____
_____

Ask any successful athlete, and they will tell you that most of their success comes from the mental preparation for training and sports events. You must believe in yourself and the power that you have to change for the better, whether it's treating a disease or whether it is to lose twenty pounds or eighty pounds; the power of belief that you can do it is vital, because it will vitalize you.

Remember to see and hear and feel your goals. Be flexible and change and improve your goals continually so that you are getting better and better.

One more point that I learned from Dr. Richard Bandler and John La Valle was, whenever dealing with a problem, ask, "Who is the greatest controlling element in my life?"

You will understand this question easily if *you* are. So take control and learn more about how to melt away the fat and build muscle. Keep in mind that mentally you want to be strong throughout this whole process. Start with your mind, and the body will follow.

Last, I came across a really good app for my iPhone/iPad that helps to lock in quickly into a meditative state. It's called Altered States. It's a selection of ambient natural noises with an induction brain-wave pattern. It helps to stimulate or sedate the nervous system and brain and puts you in control of the desired state of mind. It is available at:

http://www.banzailabs.com/brainwaveapps.html

THE KNOWLEDGE

Glycemic Index of Selected Foods

What follows is a shopping list of foods and their glycemic index. Those carbohydrates above the GI of 50–60 require some insulin or pancreatic involvement, which causes storage of the sugar as fat. Whereas slow carbohydrates with a GI of between 10 and 50 will encourage better usage of the energy and help balance the weight. Combining the carbohydrates with a good portion of protein and vegetables will cause the glycemic load to slow down.

Protein—Proteins must be chosen according to paleo-blood-type theory, and preferably they should be organic and free from hormones/antibiotics.

- Beef
- Chicken
- Turkey
- Ostrich
- Cornish hens
- Eggs
- Rabbit
- Fish
- Lamb and mutton

Dairy—Consider using organic sources and follow the blood-type rules for dairy, as it is considered a protein. Apply blood-type rules well, for example only B and AB are allowed cow's milk, and O blood must use dairy sparingly.

- Butter, ghee
- Goat's cheese
- Feta cheese
- Mozzarella
- Ricotta
- Yogurt (live acidophilus)
- Cottage cheese
- Milk (organic cows or goats)
- Milk-like beverages (almond, rice)

Vegetables—Most vegetables are of low GI values between 15 and 30. Wash vegetables before consuming.

- Arugula (10)
- Artichoke (20)
- Asparagus (15)
- Avocado (10)
- Bamboo (20)
- Bok choy (15)
- Broccoli (15)
- Brussels sprouts (15)
- Cauliflower (15)
- Courgettes (zucchini) (15)
- Celery (15)
- Chicory, endive (10)
- Chives (5–10)
- Christophene (30–35)
- Collards (20)
- Cilantro (1)
- Cucumbers (15)
- Garlic (30)
- Hearts of palm (20)
- Kale (15–20)
- Lettuce (15)
- Okra (20)
- Olives (15)
- Onions (15)
- Parsley (5)
- Peppers (10–15)
- Squash (75)
- Pumpkin (75)
- Spinach (15)
- Tomatoes (30)
- Sun-dried tomatoes (35)
- Water chestnut (60)
- Watercress (10)

Carbohydrates—If one is confident that there is no yeast activity in the body, then one can choose a slightly higher-GI food in order to supply more glucose for the upcoming workout or training session of physical activity.

- Carrots (16–33)
- Cassava/yucca (46–50)
- Black-eyed peas (38–52)
- Green peas (48–50)
- Parsnips/boiled (52)
- Yams (36–50)
- Sweet potatoes (50–54)
- Brown rice (55)
- Baked beans (48)
- Kidney beans (23–52)
- Chickpeas (36–38)
- Turnips (9)

Fruits—Always wash and clean the fruit before consuming. Once again a higher-GI fruit will supply good energy for a boosted workout from the extra sugar in the system. Only eat lower-GI fruits if one is sedentary after eating the fruit. Higher-GI fruits require vigorous exercise to burn off the sugar and fat.

- Green apples (35–38)
- Grapes (42–46)
- Bananas (52–54)
- Cherries (22)
- Pink grapefruits (25)
- Lemons (v. low)
- Limes (v. low)
- Blueberries (40–50)
- Blackberries (40–50)
- Boysenberries (40-50)
- Raspberries (40–50)
- Strawberries (40)
- Apricots (35–38)
- Pears (38)
- Plums (39)
- Peaches (40–42)
- Mangos (41–56)
- Pineapple (51)
- Honey (60)

Herbs and Other Foods—In order to ensure that there is enough variety in the diet, other miscellaneous allowable food and beverage items have been listed in the interest of clarity. Herbs, spices, and other natural flavorings have no calories, so make sure you make the meals tasty and full of flavor. It's much more satisfying to eat a little flavorful food than large amounts of food with no flavor!

- Honey (60)
- Pure chocolate/cocoa >85% (20)
- Xylitol / xylose sugar (7)
- Olive oil (0)
- Cassava fiber (30–35)
- Hummus (30)
- Almonds (15)
- Hazelnut (15)
- Macadamias (20–25)
- Curry (0)
- Black pepper (0)
- Tomato sauce (30)
- Cayenne (0)
- Oregano (1)
- Vanilla (0)
- Mustard (30–35)
- Paprika (0)
- Dill (0)
- Basil (0)
- Sage (0)
- Basil (0)
- Ginger (0)
- Ezekiel bread (35)

Beverages

- Almond Milk (30)
- Carrot juice (45)
- Coconut milk (30)
- Soy milk (30)

- Vegetable juice (35–40)
- Apple juice (42)
- Soda water (0)
- Green tea (5–10)
- Organic coffee (0)

Danger Foods with High GIs—Keep away from these foods, as they will just turn into fat. It is far better to avoid these foods completely, as they all create high insulin swings.

- Corn syrup (115–120)
- Corn flakes (85)
- Popcorn (85)
- Glucose (100)
- White sugar (75–80)
- Fried potatoes (95–100)
- Beer (100)
- Soft drinks (70)
- Doughnuts (75–90)
- Bagels (70)
- Croissants (70)
- Biscuits (70)
- French fries (54–75)
- Watermelon (75–90)
- White bread (90)
- Brown bread (65–80)
- Whole-grain bread (65)
- Rice milk (65)
- Wheat (70–80)
- Watermelon (90–110)

Snacks—Humans benefit from snacking in small amounts in between meals, as this helps to maintain optimal blood-sugar levels. Variety and moderation are key to the success of the program, as is an open mind, as you will be educating your body to a new variety of snacks.

- Yogurt with cinnamon or vanilla essence and almond flakes (45–50)
- Home-made chocolate cassava/yucca/yucca crackers with flaked almonds (35–40)
- Selected low-GI fruits, chopped and served with some cream and xylitol (30–50)
- Celery sticks with tuna (25–30)
- Celery sticks with cheese and olives (30)
- Avocado slices topped with melted cheese (25–30)
- Guacamole dip with cassava-fiber crackers (25–30)

- Cassava/yucca crackers with melted mozzarella, garlic, and tomatoes (40–45)
- Cassava/yucca chocolate biscuit (50)
- Protein—nuts, cuts of cold meats, chicken drumstick, turkey slices

Blood Chemistry Interpretation Charts

TEST	OPTIMAL RANGES HIGH - LOW	POSSIBLE CAUSES	CORRECTIVE TREATMENT
ALT	ALANINE AMINO TRANSFERASE 10 - 30 U/L	LIVER ISSUES, EXCESSIVE MUSCLE BREAKDOWN OR TURNOVER, B6 DEFICIENCY, ALCOHOLISM	MILK THISTLE, B VITAMINS, GLUTAMINE, EGGS, A VERY HEALTHY DIET.
ALB	ALBUMIN 4.0 - 5.0 g/dL	DEHYDRATION, THYROID & ADRENAL HYPO-FUNCTION, LOW STOMACH ACID, LIVER DYSFUNCTION, VITAMIN C NEED	DIGESTIVE ENZYMES, GOOD HYGIENE, EGG WHITES, ZINC, VITAMIN C.
ALP	ALKALINE PHOSPHATASE 70 - 100 U/L	BILLARY OBSTRUCTION, LIVER CELL DAMAGE, BONE LOSS, GROWTH & REPAIR, LEAKY GUT. ZINC DEFICIENCY, BIRTH CONTROL PILLS, CORTICOSTEROIDS & HORMONE REPLACEMENT THERAPY.	ZINC & FAT DIGESTION ENZYMES, MILK THISTLE, INCREASE PROTEIN CONSUMPTION (EGGS & SALMON), B VITAMINS, BROCCOLI, PUMPKIN, ASPARAGUS. A VERY HEALTHY DIET.
AMY	AMYLASE 60 - 100 mg/d1	PANCREATITIS. DAMAGE DUE TO AMYLASE PRODUCING CELLS IN PANCREAS.	CHROMIUM, PANCREATIN ENZYMES, AMYLASE ENZYMES, BROCCOLI, GRAPE JUICE, ROYAL JELLY, B5.
AST	ASPARTATE AMINOTRANFERASE 10 - 30 U/L	DEVELOPING CONGESTIVE HEAT PICTURE. CARDIOVASCULAR DYSFUNCTION, ACUTE MYOCARDIAL INFARCTION, LIVER ISSUES, EXCESSIVE MUSCLE BREAKDOWN, B6 DEFICIENCY, ALCOHOLISM.	B6 & B COMPLEX, CoQ10 (HIGH DOSES), MAGNESIUM, CALCIUM, POTASSIUM, VITAMINS A, C & E, GLUTAMINE, INCREASE PROTEIN INTAKE, A VERY HEALTHY DIET.
CA++	CALCIUM 9.2 - 10 mg/dL	HYPER-PARATHYROIDISM, HYPOTHYROIDISM, IMPAIRED CELL MEMBRANE HEALTH. CA NEEDED OR ONE OF ITS COFACTORS. LOW STOMACH ACID, LOW ALBUMIN.	BETAINE, HC1, SARDINES WITH BONES, SALMON, HERRING, LIVER, VITAMIN D, SUNSHINE, ESSENTIAL FATTY ACIDS, BROCCOLI, ASPARAGUS.
GGT	GAMMA GLUTAMIL TRANSFERASE 10 - 30 U/L	BILLARY OBSTRUCTION, LIVER CELL DAMAGE, EXCESSIVE ALCOHOL. B6 DEFICIENCY, MG NEEDED, KIDNEY FAILURE.	B6 & B COMPLEX, MAGNESIUM, GLUTAMINE, EGGS, CARROTS, AVOCADOS, A VERY HEALTHY DIET.
CRE	CREATININE 0.8 - 1.1 mg/dL	URINARY TRACT CONGESTION/ OBSTRUCTION, RENAL DYSFUNCTION, DRUGS. MUSCLE ATROPHY, NERVE/ MUSCLE DEGENERATION, MS, LIVER DISEASE, NEED FOR EXERCISE.	B COMPLEX, MAGNESIUM, POTASSIUM, VITAMIN D, PHOSPHORUS, BROCCOLI, PUMPKIN, ASPARAGUS. CHECK IRON LEVELS AND RULE OUT ANAEMIA, LOW ACIDITY DIET.

BLOOD CHEMISTRY INTERPRETATION CHARTS

TEST	OPTIMAL RANGES HIGH - LOW	POSSIBLE CAUSES	CORRECTIVE TREATMENT
GLU	GLUCOSE 80 - 100 mg/dL	INSULIN RESISTANCE & GLUCOSE INTOLERANCE, HYPOGLYCEMIA, THIAMINE NEED, ACUTE STRESS, LIVER CONGESTION, OBESITY, ACUTE PANCREATITIS, SUGAR OVERLOAD. ADULT & JUVENILE DIABETES, MELLITUS & HYPOGLYCEMIA, HYPERINSULINISM, ADRENAL HYPO FUNCTION, ALCOHOL, LIVER DAMAGE, PITUITARY HYPOFUNCTION.	CHRONIUM, MAGNESIUM, MILK THISTLE, COQ10, ESSENTIAL FATTY ACIDS, LIPOLIC ACID, LOW CARB DIET, REDUCE SUGAR CONSUMPTION. USE XYLOSE AS A REPLACEMENT.
TBIL	TOTAL BILLIRUBIN 0.2 - 1.0 mg/dL	BILLARY STASIS OR OBSTRUCTION, THYMUS DYSFUNCTION, RBC HEMOYSIS, SUGAR OVERLOAD. SPLEEN INSUFFICIENCY.	FAT DIGESTIVE ENZYMES, VITAMIN C, MYCELIZED A & E, ZINC, GLUTAMINE (DISSOLVES GALLSTONES), SERIOUSLY REDUCE SUGAR CONSUMPTION, A VERY HEALTHY DIET.
TP	TOTAL PROTEIN 6.9 - 7.4 g/dL	DEHYDRATION, LOW STOMACH ACID, LIVER DYSFUNCTION, MALNUTRITION.	WATER, ZINC, MILK THISTLE, DIGESTIVE ENZYMES.
BUN	BLOOD UREA NITROGEN 10 -16 mg/dL	RENAL DISEASE/INSUFFICIENCY, DEHYDRATION, LOW STOMACH ACID, EDEMA. LOW PROTEIN DIET, MALABSORPTION, PANCREATIC & LIVER ISSUES.	KIDNEY EXTRACT, B COMPLEX, MAGNESIUM, POTASSIUM, CALCIUM, DIGESTIVE ENZYMES, MILK THISTLE, TUMERIC, LOW ACIDITY DIET.
UA	URIC ACID 3.0 - 5.5	GOUT, YEAST & FUNGUS. ATHEROSCLEROSIS, RHEUMATOID ARTHRITIS, RENAL INSUFFICIENCY/ DISEASE, LEAKY GUT SYNDROME, DIURETICS. MOLYBDENUM, COPPER AND/OR FOLATE DEFICIENCY, PREGNANCY, CORTICOSTEROIDS, HEAVY METAL POISONING, OCCUPATIONAL HAZARDS.	MAGNESIUM, SARSAPARILLA, B COMPLEX, FOLIC ACID & ORGANIC LITHIUM, NETTLE TEA, LOW LEVELS = COPPER DEFICIENCY. USE THE DIRECTION OF A PHYSICIAN. GO ON THE STEP 1 DIET (THE HIDDEN CURE BOOK) AS HIGH URIC ACID CAN BE CAUSED BY YEAST

Basic Metabolic Panel

TEST	OPTIMAL RANGES	POSSIBLE CAUSES	POSSIBLE TREATMENTS
Ca	CALCIUM 9.2 - 10 MG/DL	HYPERPARATHYROIDISM, HYPOPARATHYROIDISM, IMPAIRED CELL MEMBRANE HEALTH. CALCIUM NEEDED OR ONE OF ITS COFACTORS, LOW STOMACH ACID, LOW ALBUMIN.	BETAINE HC1, SARDINES WITH BONES, SALMON, HERRING, LIVER, VITAMIN D, SUNSHINE, ESSENTIAL FATTY ACIDS BROCCOLI, ASPARAGUS.
CL	CHLORIDE 100 - 106 meg/L	METABOLIC ACIDOSIS, ADRENAL HYPER FUNCTION DEHYDRATION, HYPERPARATHYROIDISM, EXCESS SALT CONSUMPTION, PROLONGED DIARRHOEA & VOMITING, OVER HYDRATION, RENAL DYSFUNCTION, ADRENAL HYPO FUNCTION, CONSTIPATION.	TOO LITTLE OR TOO MUCH SEA SALT. DEHYDRATION, ADRENAL SUPPORT, DIGESTIVE ENZYMES, ELECTROLYTES.
CRE	CREATININE 0.8 - 1.1 mg/dL	URINARY TRACT CONGESTION/OBSTRUCTION, RENAL DYSFUNCTION, DRUGS. MUSCLE ATROPHY, NERVE/MUSCLE DEGENERATION, MS, LIVER DISEASE, NEED FOR EXERCISE.	B COMPLEX, MAGNESIUM, POTASSIUM, VITAMIN D, PHOSPHORUS, BROCCOLI, PUMPKIN, ASPARAGUS, CHECK IRON LEVELS AND RULE OUT ANAEMIA.
LD	LACTATED HYDROGENASE 140 - 200 U/L	LIVER DISEASE, ACUTE LIVER HEPATITIS, CIRRHOSIS, CARDIAC DISEASES, MYOCARDIAL INFARCTION AND TISSUE ALTERATIONS OF THE HEART, KIDNEY, LIVER & MUSCLE LYMPHOMA, CANCER, LEUKAEMIA, REACTIVE HYPOGLYCAEMIA, SOME DRUGS.	MILK THISTLE, SELENIUM, GARLIC & ANTI FUNGAL, CoQ10, B COMPLEX, CHECK THYROID FUNCTION, RULE OUT NEOPLASM.
MG	MAGNESIUM 2.0 - 2.3 mg/dL	RENAL DYSFUNCTION, THYROID HYPOFUNCTION, EXCESS MAGNESIUM CONTAINING ANTACIDS, DEHYDRATION, EPILEPSY, MUSCLE SPASM, ADRENAL HYPERFUNCTION, MALABSORPTION	GREEN LEAFY VEGETABLES, MAGNESIUM SUPPLEMENTS, SUPPORT KIDNEYS, LOW ACIDITY DIET.
K+	POTASSIUM 4.- 4.5 meg/L	ADRENAL HYPOFUNCTION, DEHYDRATION, TISSUE DESTRUCTION, RENAL FAILURE. ADRENAL HYPER FUNCTION, DIURETICS, ESSENTIAL HYPERTENSION, DIARRHOEA.	SUPPORT ADRENALS, REDUCE STRESS, LAUGH, MEDITATE, GET IN TOUCH WITH NATURE.
Na+	SODIUM 135 142 meg/L	ADRENAL HYPERFUNCTION, DEHYDRATION, CUSHING'S DISEASE, ADRENAL HYPOFUNCTION, ADDISON'S DISEASE, EDEMA	SUPPORT ADRENALS, REDUCE STRESS, LAUGH, MEDITATE, GET IN TOUCH WITH NATURE, DHEA THERAPY, LIQUORICE, GINSENG
T CO2	TOTAL CARBON DIOXIDE 25 - 30 meg/L	METABOLIC ALKALOSIS, RESPIRATORY ACIDOSIS. METABOLIC ACIDOSIS, RESPIRATORY ALKALOSIS	REDUCE ANTACIDS, ADJUST CALCIUM, EAT SOME ACIDIC FOODS

BLOOD SUGAR TESTING CHART

Test	Definition	Optimal Ranges mg/dL High to Low	Possible Causes	Possible Treatments
Chol	Cholesterol	150 - 220	Primary hypothyroidism, Adrenal burn out, Adrenal cortical dysfunction, Anterior pituitary hypo function, Cardiovascular disease, Atherosclerosis, Bilary status Fatty liver, Early stage Diabetes, Multiple Sclerosis	Oxidative stress and free radical activity, Heavy metal/chemical overload, LiverBiliary dysfunction, Insufficient fat intake, Vegetarian diet, Thyroid hyper function, Autoimmune processes, Adrenal hyper function.
HDL	High Density Lipo Protein Cholesterol	>55	Autoimmune processes, Hypothyroidism, Insulin use, Excess Alcohol consumption	Hyperlipide mia and atherosclerosis, Syndrome X, Oxidative stress, Heavy metal/chemical overload, Fatty liver, Lack of exercise, Hyperthyroidism.
TRIG	Triglycerides	70 -110	Syndrome X, Fatty liver, Early stage insulin resistance, CVD, Leptin Resistance, Atherosclerosis, Poor metabolism & utilisation of fats, Early stage diabetes, Adrenal cortical dysfunction, Alcoholism	Liver dysfunction, Thyroid hyper function, Autoimmune processes, Adrenal Hyperfunction
TC/H	Total cholesterol to HDL ratio		Greater proportion of VLDL & LDL compared to HDL making up total cholesterol	Greater amount of HDL compared to LDL & VLDL making up total cholesterol volume
LDL	Low density lipoprotein cholesterol	<120	Diet high in refined carbohydrates, Syndrome X, Atherosclerosis, Hyperlipidemia, Oxidative stress, Fatty Liver	Low levels of LDL reduce the risks for these diseases/dysfunction
VLDL	Very low density lipoprotein cholesterol	<30	Coronary artery disease	Low levels of VLDL reduce the risks for coronary artery disease

BLOOD SUGAR TESTING RECORD

	AM	AM	AM	LUNCH	LUNCH	DINNER	DINNER	PM	
	Waking	Before B'fast	Hour After B'fast	Before Lunch	Hour After Lunch	Before Dinner	Hour After Dinner	Bedtime	Comments
Mon									
Tues									
Wed									
Thurs									
Fri									
Sat									
Sun									

APPENDIX

Useful Contacts

For lab testing of the adrenals, sex hormones, and allergies. They both run an excellent service and test kits and reports are posted via post and email.

Genova Diagnostic

Laboratory (Allergies, hormones and Stool) 63 Zillicoa St
Asheville, NC 28801-1074 828-253-0621
800-522-4762
Fax: 828-252-9303
http://www.gdx.net
Email: cs@gsdl.com www.gsdl.com

Biohealth Labs, California, USA (Adrenal Testing and Stool)
http://biohealthlab.com/contact
800-570-2000 or 307-426-5060

For Ordering vitamins, Pregnenolone, DHEA, or adrenal glandular remedies, visit the Maas Clinic website: www.themaasclinic.com. Click the tab for Maas Store and register yourself as a patient of mine on the Store page using Reg code **LM:407**.

Make sure you use an international courier if you want to start the program early.

Watch out for our new health app coming in late 2014—to help you figure out what's going on using your latest blood-chemistry scores and physiology.

Sign up on our Facebook and Twitter pages to receive the best health tips.

About the Author

Mr. Laurens Maas
B.Sc. Ost., Dl. Hom. G.Os.C. & FBIH (UK)

Laurens Maas is a board-certified, registered osteopath, homeopath, and Functional Diagnostic Medical practitioner trained in the United Kingdom and United States. He has been practicing holistic medicine since 1993 on the Caribbean island of Barbados and the United Kingdom. He is currently studying for his US doctorate in Integrated Medicine.

The gem of the Lesser Antilles, Barbados, has a disproportionately high rate of obesity amongst the local population. Laurens Maas has consulted with and treated thousands of patients using the techniques outlined in this book. Hundreds of international clients fly in from all over the world every year specifically to be treated by Laurens using state-of-the-art Functional Diagnostic Medicine (FDM), as explained in his first and second books, *The Hidden Cure* and *Curing Diabetes [T2] in Seven Steps*.

Laurens is celebrated across the Caribbean for his unique medical mind. He solves many puzzling disease cases by drawing upon the power of a holistic approach. Laurens' treatment and diagnostic processes include conventional laboratory blood-chemistry analysis, hormone testing, terrain analysis, and microbiology and diet modification.

Creating a mega fat burn using a Functional Medicine solution, he is of the opinion that there is no need to hurt your body and mind in the quest for effective weight management.